ORTHOPEDIC CLINICS OF NORTH AMERICA

www.orthopedic.theclinics.com

Obesity

July 2018 • Volume 49 • Number 3

ELSEVIER

1600 John F. Kennedy Boulevard • Suite 1800 • Philadelphia, Pennsylvania, 19103-2899.

http://www.orthopedic.theclinics.com

ORTHOPEDIC CLINICS OF NORTH AMERICA Volume 49, Number 3
July 2018 ISSN 0030-5898, ISBN-13: 978-0-323-61068-1

Editor: Lauren Boyle
Developmental Editor: Kristen Helm

Orthopedic Clinics of North America (ISSN 0030-5898) is published quarterly by Elsevier Inc., 360 Park Avenue South, New York, NY 10010-1710. Months of issue are January, April, July, and October. Business and Editorial Offices: 1600 John F. Kennedy Blvd., Suite 1800, Philadelphia, PA 19103-2899. Customer Service Office: 3251 Riverport Lane, Maryland Heights, MO 63043. Periodicals postage paid at New York, NY and additional mailing offices. Subscription prices are $332.00 per year for (US individuals), $713.00 per year for (US institutions), $391.00 per year (Canadian individuals), $870.00 per year (Canadian institutions), $464.00 per year (international individuals), $870.00 per year (international institutions), $100.00 per year (US students), $220.00 per year (Canadian and international students). Foreign air speed delivery is included in all *Clinics* subscription prices. All prices are subject to change without notice. **POSTMASTER:** Send change of address to *Orthopedic Clinics of North America*, **Elsevier Health Sciences Division, Subscription Customer Service, 3251 Riverport Lane, Maryland Heights, MO 63043. Customer Service (orders, claims, online, change of address): Elsevier Health Sciences Division, Subscription Customer Service, 3251 Riverport Lane, Maryland Heights, MO 63043. Tel: 1-800-654-2452 (U.S. and Canada); 314-447-8871 (outside U.S. and Canada). Fax: 314-447-8029. E-mail:** journalscustomerservice-usa@elsevier.com **(for print support);** journalsonlinesupport-usa@elsevier.com **(for online support).**

Reprints. For copies of 100 or more, of articles in this publication, please contact the Commercial Reprints Department, Elsevier Inc., 360 Park Avenue South, New York, NY 10010-1710. Tel.: 212-633-3874; Fax: 212-633-3820; E-mail: reprints@elsevier.com.

Orthopedic Clinics of North America is covered in *MEDLINE/PubMed* (*Index Medicus*), *Cinahl, Excerpta Medica,* and *Cumulative Index to Nursing and Allied Health Literature.*

PROGRAM OBJECTIVE

Orthopedic Clinics of North America offers clinical review articles on the most cutting-edge technologies and techniques in the field, including knee and hip reconstruction, hand and wrist, pediatrics, trauma, shoulder and elbow, and foot and ankle.

TARGET AUDIENCE

Practicing orthopedic surgeons, orthopedic residents, and other healthcare professionals who specialize in orthopedic technologies and techniques for knee and hip reconstruction, hand and wrist, pediatrics, trauma, shoulder and elbow, and foot and ankle.

LEARNING OBJECTIVES

Upon completion of this activity, participants will be able to:
1. Review the role of bariatric surgery in the obese total joint arthroplasty patient.
2. Discuss obesity in pediatric trauma.
3. Recognize the impact of obesity on orthopaedic upper extremity surgery.

ACCREDITATION

The Elsevier Office of Continuing Medical Education (EOCME) is accredited by the Accreditation Council for Continuing Medical Education (ACCME) to provide continuing medical education for physicians.

The EOCME designates this enduring material for a maximum of 15 *AMA PRA Category 1 Credit*(s)™. Physicians should claim only the credit commensurate with the extent of their participation in the activity.

All other healthcare professionals requesting continuing education credit for this enduring material will be issued a certificate of participation.

DISCLOSURE OF CONFLICTS OF INTEREST

The EOCME assesses conflict of interest with its instructors, faculty, planners, and other individuals who are in a position to control the content of CME activities. All relevant conflicts of interest that are identified are thoroughly vetted by EOCME for fair balance, scientific objectivity, and patient care recommendations. EOCME is committed to providing its learners with CME activities that promote improvements or quality in healthcare and not a specific proprietary business or a commercial interest.

The planning committee, staff, authors and editors listed below have identified no financial relationships or relationships to products or devices they or their spouse/life partner have with commercial interest related to the content of this CME activity:
Philip Ashley, MD; Frederick M. Azar, MD; Michael J. Beebe, MD; Clayton C. Bettin, MD; Jared S. Bookman, MD; Lauren Boyle; James H. Calandruccio, MD; Michael J. Conklin, MD; Jon Cooper Wall, Jr, MD; Kay Daugherty; Ivan De Martino, MD; Ajit J. Deshmukh, MD; Shawn R. Gilbert, MD; Lawrence V. Gulotta, MD; Aaron J. Guyer, MD; Mario Hevesi, MD; Jessica M. Hooper, MD; R. Miles Hulick, MD; Richard Iorio, MD; Alison Kemp; Brendan J. MacKay, MD; Benjamin M. Mauck, MD; Bradley O. Osemwengie, BS; Jeffrey M. Pearson, MD; Hillary Powers Wall, BS; Kevin F. Purcell, MD; Parthiv Rathod, MD; Ran Schwarzkopf, MD, MSc; Clay A. Spitler, MD; Matthew Stewart, MD; Jeyanthi Surendrakumar.

The planning committee, staff, authors and editors listed below have identified financial relationships or relationships to products or devices they or their spouse/life partner have with commercial interest related to the content of this CME activity:
Patrick F. Bergin, MD: is a consultant/advisor for Acumed, A Colson Associate and Depuy Synthes.
Matthew L. Graves, MD: has participated in a speaker's bureau and acted as a consultant and/or advisor for DePuy Synthes.
Benjamin J. Grear, MD: has received royalties from Elsevier, Inc.
William M. Mihalko, MD: has participated in a speakers' bureau for Aesculap, Inc. - a B. Braun company and CeramTec GmbH; has received research support from the United States Depaartment of Defense and Stryker; has served as a consultant/advisor for Zimmer Biomet; and receives royalties from Elsevier, Inc.
Mark E. Morrey, MD: owns stock in Tenex.
George V. Russell, MD: owns stock in SMV Scientific and Zimmer Biomet.
Jeffrey R. Sawyer, MD: has participated in a speakers' bureau for DePuy Synthes and NuVasive, Inc. and receives royalties from Elsevier, Inc. and Wolters Kluwer.
Thomas (Quin) Throckmorton, MD: has participated in a speakers' bureau for Zimmer Biomet, owns stock in Gilead, and receives royalties from Elsevier, Inc.
Patrick C. Toy, MD: has been a consultant/advisor for Zimmer Biomet, Medtronic, and Smith & Nephew. He also receives royalties and/or holds patents with Innomed, Inc.
John C. Weinlein, MD: receives royalties from Elsevier, Inc.

UNAPPROVED/OFF-LABEL USE DISCLOSURE

The EOCME requires CME faculty to disclose to the participants:
1. When products or procedures being discussed are off-label, unlabelled, experimental, and/or investigational (not US Food and Drug Administration [FDA] approved); and
2. Any limitations on the information presented, such as data that are preliminary or that represent ongoing research, interim analyses, and/or unsupported opinions. Faculty may discuss information about pharmaceutical agents that is outside of FDA-approved labelling. This information is intended solely for CME and is not intended to promote off-label use of these

medications. If you have any questions, contact the medical affairs department of the manufacturer for the most recent prescribing information.

TO ENROLL

To enroll in the *Orthopedic Clinics of North America* Continuing Medical Education program, call customer service at 1-800-654-2452 or sign up online at http://www.theclinics.com/home/cme. The CME program is available to subscribers for an additional annual fee of USD 215.

METHOD OF PARTICIPATION

In order to claim credit, participants must complete the following:
1. Complete enrolment as indicated above.
2. Read the activity.
3. Complete the CME Test and Evaluation. Participants must achieve a score of 70% on the test. All CME Tests and Evaluations must be completed online.

CME INQUIRIES/SPECIAL NEEDS

For all CME inquiries or special needs, please contact elsevierCME@elsevier.com.

EDITORIAL BOARD

CONTRIBUTORS

AUTHORS

PHILIP ASHLEY, MD
Assistant Professor, Department of
Orthopaedic Surgery, The University of
Alabama at Birmingham, Birmingham,
Alabama

PATRICK F. BERGIN, MD
Associate Professor, Department of
Orthopaedic Surgery and Rehabilitation,
The University of Mississippi Medical
Center, Jackson, Mississippi

JARED S. BOOKMAN, MD
Department of Orthopedic Surgery, NYU
School of Medicine, NYU Langone Health,
NYU Langone Orthopedic Hospital,
New York, New York

MICHAEL J. CONKLIN, MD
Department of Orthopedic Surgery, Doctor
of Medicine, University of Cincinnati,
Pediatric Orthopedic Surgeon, Associate
Professor, UAB School of Medicine,
Children's of Alabama, Birmingham,
Alabama

IVAN DE MARTINO, MD
Clinical Fellow, Sports and Shoulder Service,
Hospital for Special Surgery, New York,
New York

AJIT J. DESHMUKH, MD
Assistant Professor, Departments of Adult
Reconstruction and Orthopedic Surgery,
NYU School of Medicine, NYU Langone
Health, NYU Langone Orthopedic Hospital,
New York, New York

SHAWN R. GILBERT, MD
Professor, Department of
Orthopaedic Surgery, The University
of Alabama at Birmingham,
Birmingham, Alabama

MATTHEW L. GRAVES, MD
Professor, Department of Orthopaedic, The
University of Mississippi Medical Center,
Jackson, Mississippi

LAWRENCE V. GULOTTA, MD
Associate Attending Orthopedic Surgeon,
Sports and Shoulder Service, Hospital for
Special Surgery, Associate Professor of
Orthopaedic Surgery, Weill Cornell Medicine,
New York, New York

AARON J. GUYER, MD
Tallahassee Orthopedic Clinic, Clinical
Assistant Professor in Surgery, Florida State
University College of Medicine, Tallahassee,
Florida; Clinical Faculty, Alabama College of
Osteopathic Medicine, Dothan, Alabama;
Chief of Orthopedic Surgery, Tallahassee
Memorial HealthCare, Tallahassee, Florida

MARIO HEVESI, MD
Mayo Clinic, Rochester, Minnesota

JESSICA M. HOOPER, MD
Resident Physician, Department of
Orthopaedic Surgery, NYU Langone
Orthopaedic Hospital, New York, New York

R. MILES HULICK, MD
Department of Orthopaedic Surgery, The
University of Mississippi Medical Center,
Jackson, Mississippi

RICHARD IORIO, MD
Department of Orthopedic Surgery, NYU
School of Medicine, NYU Langone Health,
NYU Langone Orthopedic Hospital,
New York, New York

BRENDAN J. MacKAY, MD
Assistant Professor, Department of
Orthopaedic Surgery, Texas Tech University
Health Sciences Center, Lubbock, Texas;
Diplomate, American Board of Orthopaedic
Surgeons; Fellow, American Academy of
Orthopaedic Surgeons; Subspecialty
Certificate in Orthopaedic Surgery of the
Hand, Candidate Member, American Society
for Surgery of the Hand; Member, American
Association of Hand Surgery, Director of Hand
and Microvascular Surgery, UMC Health
System, Lubbock, Texas

MARK E. MORREY, MD
Mayo Clinic, Rochester, Minnesota

BRADLEY O. OSEMWENGIE, BS
Medical Student, Texas Tech University Health
Sciences Center, School of Medicine,
Lubbock, Texas

JEFFREY M. PEARSON, MD
Department of Orthopedic Surgery,
Doctor of Medicine, Louisiana State
University, PGY3 Orthopedic
Surgery Resident, UAB School
of Medicine, Children's of Alabama,
Birmingham, Alabama

KEVIN F. PURCELL, MD
House Officer, Department of Orthopaedic
Surgery and Rehabilitation, The University of
Mississippi Medical Center, Jackson,
Mississippi

PARTHIV RATHOD, MD
Department of Orthopedic Surgery, NYU
School of Medicine, NYU Langone Health,
NYU Langone Orthopedic Hospital,
New York, New York

GEORGE V. RUSSELL, MD
Professor and Chairman, Department of
Orthopaedic Surgery, The University of
Mississippi Medical Center, Jackson, Mississippi

RAN SCHWARZKOPF, MD, MSc
Associate Professor, Adult Reconstructive
Surgery, Department of Adult Reconstruction,
NYU Langone Orthopaedic Hospital,
New York, New York

CLAY A. SPITLER, MD
Assistant Professor, Department of
Orthopaedic Surgery, The University of
Mississippi Medical Center, Jackson,
Mississippi

MATTHEW STEWART, MD
The Hughston Clinic, Columbus, Georgia

HILLARY POWERS WALL, BS
Medical Student, Texas Tech University Health
Sciences Center, School of Medicine,
Lubbock, Texas

JON COOPER WALL Jr, MD
Resident Physician, Department of
Orthopaedic Surgery, Texas Tech University
Health Sciences Center, Lubbock, Texas

CONTENTS

Knee and Hip Reconstruction
Patrick C. Toy and William M. Mihalko

Obesity is an epidemic in our healthcare system. Obesity poses several challenges and raises unique issues for the arthroplasty surgeon. Obese patients
are at higher risk for infection and dislocation. Additionally, obese patients
have poorer implant survivorship and functional scores post-operatively.
Obesity is a modifiable risk factor, and weight loss preoperatively should be
strongly considered. Obese patients must be counseled so that they have realistic expectations after total joint arthroplasty.

Though bariatric surgery is a proven means of weight loss and treatment for
obesity-related comorbidities in morbidly obese patients, it is not yet clear how
it affects outcomes after total joint arthroplasty in this high-risk patient population.
This article explores the effects of obesity and bariatric surgery on osteoarthritis
and total joint arthroplasty, and also discusses the financial and ethical implications
of the use of bariatric surgery for risk reduction prior to total joint arthroplasty.

Trauma
John C. Weinlein and Michael J. Beebe

The rates of obesity continue to rise in the US and the overall impact of obesity
on healthcare spending and patient outcomes after trauma is considerable.
The unique physiology of the obese places them at higher risk for complications including infection, failure of fixation, nonunion, multi-organ failure, and
death. These physiologic differences and overall patient size can make orthopedic care in the obese trauma patient more difficult, but appropriate initial
resuscitation, careful preoperative planning, meticulous surgical technique,
diligent postoperative medical management, and specialized rehabilitation
give these patients their best opportunity at a good outcome.

Acetabular and pelvic ring injuries in the obese patient are difficult to treat. Obese
patients require great attention to detail during the trauma evaluation to prevent a
myriad of medical and anesthetic complications in the perioperative period. Radiographic evaluation of these patients is often compromised by modalities available
and loss of resolution with plain film imaging. Patient positioning needs to be

meticulous to ensure stability on the bed while allowing access to the operative site, preventing pressure necrosis, and minimizing ventilation pressure. Complications after surgical treatment are relatively common and are often due to infection and loss of fixation. Careful technique can mitigate but not prevent these complications.

Pediatrics
Jeffrey R. Sawyer

Obesity is a common problem in children and adolescents with neuromuscular disease. The available literature on obesity in cerebral palsy, spina bifida, and Duchenne muscular dystrophy as it relates to orthopaedic treatment is reviewed. This includes the demographics and measurement of obesity as well as the mechanisms of obesity in these individuals. In addition, the effect of obesity on function, patient evaluation, and orthopaedic treatment are reviewed.

Obese children with high energy injuries present with more severe injuries, more extremity injuries, and higher injury severity scores. They are at increased risk for complications, prolonged ventilation and ICU stays, and have increased mortality. Obesity is associated with altered bone mass accrual and higher fracture rates. Obese patients have a higher risk of loss of reduction of forearm fractures, more severe supracondylar fractures, and a higher likelihood of lateral condylar fractures. Obese patients are more likely to have complications with femoral fractures and have higher rates of foot and ankle fracture.

Hand and Wrist
Benjamin M. Mauck and James H. Calandruccio

The annual economic burden of obesity rivals that of smoking in the US. With an estimated one-third of the US population being classified as obese, it is of utmost importance for surgical hand specialists to be informed on the management considerations pertinent to these patients. These patients are associated with an increased rate of upper extremity injury, carpal tunnel syndrome, and upper extremity osteoarthritis. Preoperative medical considerations should evaluate the comorbid conditions such as cardiovascular disease, pulmonary disease, and diabetes mellitus. Intraoperative and anesthetic considerations should evaluate the need for specialized equipment, patient positioning, and the physiology specific to the obese patient. Postoperative considerations should include the increased risk of surgical site infections, malunion, and cardiovascular complications such as venous thromboembolism (VTE). After review of the literature, there are currently no direct contraindications for the obese patient to undergo an orthopaedic procedure as long as the appropriate considerations have been made. It is also suggested in current literature that surgery of the hand and upper extremity may be somewhat immune to the postoperative complications seen in other regions of the body.

OBESITY

PREFACE

Obesity

Obesity continues to be a national health problem, linked to a number of chronic medical conditions, such as diabetes and heart disease, and even to some types of cancer. The estimated annual health care costs of obesity-related illness are a staggering $190.2 billion or nearly 21% of annual medical spending in the United States. Childhood obesity alone is responsible for $14 billion in direct medical costs. Obesity has risen a full 34% since 1960, while morbid obesity is up sixfold. If the prevalence continues on the current trend, it is estimated that by 2030 almost half of the world's population will be overweight or obese.

In addition to its associated morbidities, obesity has detrimental effects on a wide variety of musculoskeletal conditions and their treatment. Many orthopedic conditions are more frequent in obese individuals than in their nonobese counterparts, and obesity also may worsen progression of these disorders, as well as negatively affect outcomes of orthopedic treatment. Authors in this issue of *Orthopedic Clinics of North America* discuss a number of orthopedic procedures in patients of all ages that are affected by obesity, from total joint arthroplasty to treatment of pediatric neuromuscular disorders.

Drs Bookman, Schwarzkoph, Rathod, Iorio, and Deshmukh emphasize the importance of obesity as a modifiable risk factor in patients undergoing total joint arthroplasty, and Drs Hooper, Deshmukh, and Schwarzkoph discuss how bariatric surgery affects total joint arthroplasty, as well as ethical and financial implications of its use. Drs De Martino and Gulotta point out that, although obesity increases the complication rate in total shoulder arthroplasty, it does not have a detrimental effect on functional outcomes nor does it increase hospital charges. The need for stronger, more durable implants for total elbow arthroplasty in obese patients is discussed by Drs Morrey and Hevesi, with emphasis on the complications and revision burden related to posttraumatic deformity and obesity.

Treatment of polytrauma in obese patients is the focus of Drs Spitler, Hulick, Graves, Russell, and Bergin's article, which notes the higher risk of complications and the difficulties in orthopedic care of obese patients. Some of those difficulties, such as radiographic evaluation and patient positioning, are discussed in the article by Drs Purcell, Bergin, Spitler, Graves, and Russell on pelvic and acetabular fractures in obese patients. These authors note that, while careful technique can mitigate complications such as infection and loss of fixation, it cannot totally prevent them.

As noted by Drs Stewart and Guyer and by Drs J. Wall, H. Wall, Osemwengie, and MacKay, obesity does not appear to be as important a factor in the outcomes of surgery of the foot/ankle or hand/wrist. However, comorbid conditions, such as cardiovascular disease, pulmonary disease, and diabetes mellitus, can have detrimental effects and should be considered.

Obesity is present in approximately 20% of children and adolescents, and in even more with neuromuscular disease. Drs Conklin and Pearson discuss the effects of obesity on function, patient evaluation, and orthopedic treatment in these patients, as well as review the measurement and mechanics of obesity. Drs Ashley and Gilbert note that obese children with high-energy injuries have more severe injuries, higher severity scores, longer ICU stays, and even increased mortality. Complications are more frequent after almost all fractures, including those of the forearm, elbow, femur, and foot and ankle.

Together, these articles give an excellent overview of how obesity affects orthopedic surgery and how orthopedic surgeons can ameliorate some of the complications associated with obesity. We hope readers will find information relevant to their practices and patients.

Frederick M. Azar, MD
Campbell Clinic
University of Tennessee–Campbell Clinic
Department of Orthopaedic Surgery
1211 Union Avenue, Suite 510
Memphis, TN 38104, USA

E-mail address:
fazar@campbellclinic.com

Orthop Clin N Am 49 (2018) xiii
https://doi.org/10.1016/j.ocl.2018.04.001
0030-5898/18/© 2018 Published by Elsevier Inc.

Knee and Hip Reconstruction

Obesity
The Modifiable Risk Factor in Total Joint Arthroplasty

Jared S. Bookman, MD*, Ran Schwarzkopf, MD, MSc,
Parthiv Rathod, MD, Richard Iorio, MD,
Ajit J. Deshmukh, MD

KEYWORDS

- Arthroplasty • Total hip arthroplasty • Total knee arthroplasty • Obesity • Risk factors

---

KEY POINTS

- Obesity is associated with increased complication rates in arthroplasty patients.
- Obese patients are at higher risk for infection and dislocation, and have poorer implant survivorship and functional scores postoperatively.
- To some degree, obesity is a modifiable risk factor and nutritional or bariatric surgery evaluation should be considered.
- Obese patients must be counseled to set realistic expectations after arthroplasty.

INTRODUCTION

Obesity is a significant and growing challenge facing the entire health care system. It has reached epidemic status in the United States. Obesity poses several challenges and raises unique issues for the arthroplasty surgeon.[1] Of the US population, 37% is classified as obese and rates are climbing.[2,3] Overall, medical costs in the United States due to obesity exceed $275 billion and account for more than 20% of all US health care expenditure.[4]

For adults, the World Health Organization defines a normal body mass index (BMI) as 19.5 to 24.9 kg/m^2 and overweight as 25 to 29.9 kg/m^2. A BMI greater than 30 kg/m^2 is defined as obese, greater than 40 kg/m^2 as morbidly obese, and greater than 50 kg/m^2 as superobese.[5] The terminology of class 1 obesity (BMI 30.0–34.9 kg/m^2), class II obesity (35.0–39.9 kg/m^2), and class III obesity (40.0 kg/m^2 and up) can also be used.[5]

The purpose of this discussion is to characterize how the modifiable risk factor of obesity interacts with total joint arthroplasty (TJA). This article examines the role obesity plays in early progression of osteoarthritis (OA) and need for TJA; discusses perioperative optimization, the role of bariatric surgery, and the rate of complications in obese patients; and assesses the outcomes of arthroplasty in obese patients.

INCIDENCE AND TIMING OF ARTHROPLASTY

It stands to reason that obese patients are at higher risk of developing OA.[6,7] OA is multifactorial in origin and obesity is among the principal modifiable risk factors.[4] The intuitive biomechanical explanation is clear: increased joint reactive forces from higher body weight cause subsequent wear and articular cartilage breakdown.[6] Obesity may also act via local and systemic biomechanical changes to activate inflammatory pathways that affect progression of cartilage damage and perception of pain.[3,6] Although OA has been labeled as noninflammatory, there

---

Disclosure Statement: See last page of article.
Department of Orthopedic Surgery, NYU School of Medicine, NYU Langone Health, NYU Langone Orthopedic Hospital, 301 East 17th Street, Suite 1402, New York, NY 10003, USA
* Corresponding author.
E-mail address: Jared.Bookman@nyumc.org

is evidence that it has an inflammatory component. Obesity is characterized by secretion of proinflammatory cytokines causing a low-grade, chronic inflammatory state that may contribute to progression of OA.[6]

Several studies have assessed the role of obesity on the timing of arthroplasty. A biomechanical model by Recnik and colleagues[7] assessed a cohort of 431 consecutive hip arthroplasty subjects. They used radiographic parameters to model peak contact hip stresses and joint reactive forces. They found that increased body weight tracked directly with increased hip contact stresses in their model. Additionally, higher body weight was significantly correlated with earlier age at total hip arthroplasty (THA).[7]

A large cohort study by Bourne and colleagues[8] of 54,406 subjects from the Canadian Joint Registry analyzed the association between obesity and the subsequent need for hip or knee arthroplasty. Compared with a control group of subjects with BMIs 25 kg/m^2 or less,[2] they found that increasing BMI was progressively correlated to higher risk of arthroplasty. At BMI 25 to 29.9 kg/m^2, risk was 3.2-fold higher for TKA and 1.92-fold higher for THA. At BMI 30 to 34.9 kg/m^2, relative risk progressed to 8.53 for total knee arthroplasty (TKA), and 3.42 for THA. At BMI 35 to 39.9, risk was 18.73 for TKA, and 5.24 for THA. Finally, for those subjects with BMI greater than 40 kg/m^2, risk was 32.73-fold higher for TKA, and 8.56-fold higher for THA. The data support the conclusion that obesity is a significant risk factor for severe OA progressing to need for arthroplasty, likely disproportionately affecting progression of knee OA more than hip OA.

In a 2011 study in *Annals of Internal Medicine*, Losina and colleagues[9] estimated the impact of obesity on various associated medical conditions. Their analysis attempted to quantify an overall loss of per-person quality-adjusted life years due to knee arthritis in obese subjects. Subjects lost 3.5 quality-adjusted life years due to knee OA from obesity, with a total of 86 million quality-adjusted life years lost in the United States due to obesity and/or knee OA. Their model demonstrated that reducing obesity to the levels of 10 years earlier could avert 111,206 knee replacements.[9]

PREOPERATIVE CONSIDERATIONS

Obesity is associated with multiple medical comorbidities that can negatively affect both the results of arthroplasty and the associated medical and anesthetic risks.[10] Diabetes, obstructive sleep apnea, and cardiopulmonary disease are all clearly associated with obesity and significantly increase risk of overall complications.[10]

Diabetes is a major complicating factor for arthroplasty. A recent study, analyzing a large cohort of morbidly obese (BMI >40 kg/m^2) subjects who underwent TKA, looked at diabetes and insulin dependence as an independent risk factor, with a cohort stratified into nondiabetics, type II diabetics who required no insulin, and type II diabetics who used insulin.[11] All subjects had complication rates far greater than the norm in nonobese subjects (74%–85% 10-year reoperation rate and 5%–9% infection rates). The nondiabetic and diabetic morbidly obese subjects had similarly high complication rates; however, the insulin-dependent diabetics had even higher complication rates, with significantly increased rates of reoperation (75% 10-year reoperation rate) and prosthetic joint infection (PJI; 9% 10-year infection rate). Overall, implant survivorship rates at 10 years (84% for insulin-dependent diabetics) were also significantly decreased.

Obstructive sleep apnea and restrictive lung disease pose multiple challenges in the perioperative period. Obesity causes a restrictive lung disease picture, which makes ventilating these patients much more difficult, with significantly decreased airway compliance.[1] Obstructive sleep apnea, of which obesity is a major risk factor, increases the risk of dangerous apneic episodes, leading to hypoxia, especially due to the use of general anesthetic agents and opiates in the perioperative period.[1] The risk screening questionnaire for obstructive sleep apnea, the STOP-BANG score, allows for a quick screening for this condition. STOP-BANG is an acronym for the screening questions: Snoring, often feeling Tired, Observed apnea, high blood Pressure, BMI greater than 35 kg/m^2, Age greater than 50, Neck circumference greater than 16 inches, and male Gender.[1] For this reason, many anesthesiologists advocate for increased use of neuraxial anesthesia and regional blocks in these high-risk patients to help make anesthesia safer.[10]

PREOPERATIVE WEIGHT LOSS AND THE ROLE OF BARIATRIC SURGERY

It is common practice to encourage weight loss in obese patients before arthroplasty.

Guidelines vary but many centers have practices to refer all morbidly obese patients to a weight loss clinic before considering THA or TKA. Strong recommendations should be made for improved diet and decreased obesity. Referral to an appropriate specialist should be made to help achieve these goals.[6]

If medical weight loss fails, bariatric surgery should also be considered. Watts and colleagues[12] performed a matched cohort study and compared the outcomes of obese THA subjects who underwent bariatric surgery preoperatively to those who did not. Mean BMIs improved from 49.7 to 35.3 in the bariatric group. Subjects in the preoperative bariatric surgery cohort were significantly less likely to require short-term reoperation (hazard ratio [HR] 3.2) or longer term revision (HR 5.4) compared with subjects who did not have bariatric surgery before the THA surgery.[12]

However, this conclusion is controversial. A meta-analysis of subjects who underwent bariatric surgery before arthroplasty, with a total of 657 bariatric surgery subjects compared with 22,691 obese control subjects, found no statistically significant differences in superficial infection, deep infection, venous thromboembolism (VTE), or revision surgery.[13]

Contrary to popular perception, a large percentage of obese patients are also malnourished.[14] In a recent review of obese patients scheduled to undergo bariatric surgery, 15% were hypoalbuminemic, 93% had vitamin D deficiencies, and 36% had iron deficiencies.[14] Hypoalbumenia, specifically, has been given particular attention because it has been associated with increased risk of postoperative complications.[1] Given the prevalence of nutritional deficiencies in these patients, even if not undergoing bariatric surgery, a nutritional evaluation is recommended to help correct these deficiencies preoperatively.

COMPLICATIONS

Infection

Obesity and increased BMI has consistently been shown to be associated with both increased early and late infection. This association has been consistently and reliably demonstrated with both THA and TKA.[15,16]

In a landmark study on the topic, Dowsey and colleagues[17] prospectively followed 1214 consecutive TKA subjects for 1 year to compare infection rates between obese and nonobese subjects. The overall infection rate was 1.5% and obese subjects were at much higher risk, with an odds ratio (OR) for a deep PJI of 8.96.

This same association has been demonstrated in multiple large registry studies.[18,19] In a retrospective cohort study of 56,216 TKA patients over an 8-year period in the Kaiser-Permanente system, it was shown that BMI greater than 35 kg/m^2 carried a hazard risk ratio of 1.47 for deep infection.[19] Similarly, a report from the New Zealand Joint Registry of 64,566 primary TKA surgeries over a 13-year period, demonstrated that the OR for revision for infection was 3.35 in patients with a BMI greater than 40 kg/m^2 when compared with those with a BMI less than 35 kg/m^2.[18]

Similar trends have been shown in THA.[18,20] A large single-specialty center retrospective review of 3672 consecutive primary THA cases demonstrated that BMI greater than 40 kg/m^2 was a significant risk factor for deep PJI, with an OR of 4.13.[20] However, a recent systematic review of complication rates in THA demonstrates that, although the association between THA and infection is clear, the magnitude is likely lower than that for TKA.[4]

Importantly, not only is obesity associated with increased risk of periprosthetic infection but an obese patient with an infected TKA is also more likely to fail a 2-stage reimplantation procedure.[21] In a 2-to-1 matched cohort study of morbidly obese subjects undergoing revision TKA, Watts and colleagues[21] demonstrated that reinfection risk following 2-stage reimplantation was 22% in the morbidly obese group versus 4% in the nonobese group (P<.01).

Total Hip Arthroplasty Dislocation Rate

Other than infection, dislocation is among the principal early complications in THA. In a series of 1617 subjects in the United Kingdom, BMI was highly correlated with increased incidence of instability. For every 10-point increase in BMI, the risk of dislocation increased by 113.9%.[22]

Elkins and colleagues[23] performed a sophisticated biomechanical analysis, developing a finite element model of a THA construct in an obese patient. In their model, they were able to adjust BMI, creating soft tissue thigh impingement. They mechanistically demonstrated that at BMI greater than 40 kg/m^2 increased soft tissue at the thigh, placed a laterally directed force on the prosthesis, and made dislocation more likely. This risk was slightly mitigated by lower cup abduction angles and higher offset necks; however, increases in head size were not protective. Huffman and colleagues[24] have similarly demonstrated, in a motion capture study, that obese subjects have significantly higher hip abduction angles and abduction movements during the sit-to stand motion. Peak hip abduction angles were 50% greater in the obese group, and the hip was much more abducted throughout the entire sit-to-stand cycle.[24]

Survivorship and Need for Revision

It stands to reason that a higher BMI patient would put higher mechanical strain on an implanted prosthesis that would lead to increased wear, shorter survivorship, and increased need for revision due to aseptic failure. Two recent large-meta analysis studies have assessed this reasoning in both TKA and THA.[25–27]

A recent large meta-analysis pooled 20 studies, for an overall group of 15,276 TKA subjects.[25] The overall revision rate in the cohort was significantly higher for obese subjects, OR 1.30.[25] However, when assessing for revisions specifically for aseptic loosening, no statistically significant difference was found. A study with 14-year follow-up assessing the results of overall implant survivorship in obese versus nonobese subjects found that implant survival was at 97% in the nonobese subject cohort, but only 93% in the obese subject cohort.[27] Abdel and colleagues[26] found a significantly higher failure rate due to aseptic tibial loosening in obese subjects with BMI greater than 35 kg/m^2 undergoing TKA, with a 15-year-risk of 2.7%. They recommended considering additional fixation, with possible stemmed primary implants in obese subjects undergoing TKA. A recent prospective cohort study by Mulhall and colleagues[28] of 291 consecutive revision TKA subjects similarly found that the majority of their revision cohort was obese and that BMI was significant risk factor for worse survivorship of primary TKA components and increased risk of progression to early revision.

With regard to THA, a similar association is found in the literature.[29,30] In a cohort of revision THA subjects at a single center, the relative risk for early revision (within 5 years) due to aseptic failure was found to be 4.7 (BMI >30). In subjects with a BMI greater than 30, aseptic failure was the cause of 56% of early revisions, significantly higher than nonobese subjects (12%).[29] In a superobese cohort with BMI greater than 50 kg/m^2, Issa and colleagues[31] found overall poor implant survivorship. They matched these subjects to a nonobese group, with a 6-year follow-up. Implant survivorship was only 89.6% in the superobese group, compared with 97.8% in the nonobese group. Meta-analysis data of 5137 THA subjects also supports this trend, with higher revision rates for aseptic loosening in subjects with a BMI greater than 30 kg/m^2 (OR 0.6 favoring less revision in nonobese subjects).[30]

Venous Thromboembolism

VTE, including deep vein thrombosis (DVT) and pulmonary embolism (PE), are common and potentially severe complications after TJA, and several studies have specifically examined the rates of VTE in obese subjects.[32,33] Friedman and colleagues[32] analyzed the Regulation of Coagulation in Orthopedic Surgery Clinical Trial data of 12,355 THA and TKA subjects and found that although morbidly obese subjects (BMI >40 kg/m^2) were at overall higher rates of adverse events, they had no significant increase in asymptomatic DVT, symptomatic DVT, or PE postoperatively.

Similarly, D'Apuzzo and colleagues[33] examined the Healthcare Cost and Utilization Project Nationwide Inpatient Sample database with 1,777,609 primary TKA cases, of which 98,410 were morbidly obese. They found no significant difference in DVT rates, with a rate of 0.44% among the morbidly obese cohort compared with a rate of 0.38% in the nonobese cohort, with an OR of 0.8 (0.7–1.0). They also found no significant difference in PE rates at 0.45% in the obese cohort as compared with 0.39% in the nonobese cohort, OR 0.8 (0.7–1.0).[33]

OUTCOMES

Because the goal of any arthroplasty operation is to reduce pain and improve function, it must also be assessed if total hip and knee arthroplasty in obese patients has similar subjective functional outcomes in this higher risk cohort. A systematic review of TKA outcomes in obesity found that Knee Society Scores were significantly better in nonobese subjects, by 3.23 points on average.[25] A meta-analysis of THA subjects showed a similar effect with postoperative Harris Hip Scores, with a mean difference of 4.54 points higher in the nonobese group.[30]

Naziri and colleagues[34] specifically looked at TKA in a cohort of superobese subjects, with BMI greater than 50 kg/m^2, which was matched to a control group of nonobese subjects. At a mean follow-up of 5 years, these subjects had lower Knee Society scores at 82 compared with 90, and achieved poorer knee flexion at 109° compared with 121°. Similar trends were shown in the same groups' cohort of THA subjects with BMI greater than 50 kg/m^2. Superobese subjects at mean 6-year follow-up had significantly lower postoperative Harris Hip Scores (82 compared with 91), Short Form Health Survey (SF)-36 scores, and University of California, Los Angeles (UCLA) activity scale scores.[31]

Although nonobese patients generally rate higher postoperative functional scores than their obese counterparts, the mean difference between preoperative and postoperative scores is often similar in these patients.[35] Chee and colleagues[35] matched obese subjects with a nonobese control cohort and found that, although postoperative Harris Hip Scores at 5 years were significantly better in the nonobese cohort (91.8 vs 85.5, $P<.05$), the mean change in score from preoperative to postoperative was similar between the groups (52.0 vs 48.1, $P = .8$). Essentially, although nonobese patients have better absolute functional scores, the relative improvement in scores from surgery may be similar between obese and nonobese patients.

SUMMARY

Overall, obesity is an extremely prevalent complicating factor that poses several challenges for the arthroplasty surgeon. Obese patients are at much higher risk for infection after THA or TKA and dislocation after THA. They also have poorer implant survivorship and lower absolute functional scores postoperatively. However, obese patients also have more severe and earlier progression of OA, and can benefit significantly from TJA.

The ethics of this issue must also be considered. Many surgeons and centers do not recommend limiting access to TJA in obese patients; however, it is common practice to refer for nutritional evaluation, medical weight loss, or bariatric evaluation preoperatively. Patients must be counseled on the increased complication risk and need to have realistic expectations of their excepted outcome postoperatively. Delaying surgery to optimize the patient and improve the chances for a good outcome is often the right thing to do for the patient, the physician, the hospital, and the payer. As obesity rates continue to grow, this is an issue that will only become more important and commonplace for the arthroplasty surgeon.

DISCLOSURE STATEMENT

The study received no funding sources. Dr J.S. Bookman, Dr P. Rathod, and Dr A.J. Deshmukh have no disclosures. Dr R. Schwarzkopf: American Academy of Orthopaedic Surgeons: board or committee member; American Association of Hip and Knee Surgeons: board or committee member; *Arthroplasty Today*: editorial or governing board; Gauss surgical: stock or stock options; Intelijoint: paid consultant, stock or stock options; *Journal of Arthroplasty*: editorial or governing board; and Smith and Nephew: paid consultant, research support. Dr R. Iorio: American Association of Hip and Knee Surgeons: board or committee member; Bioventis: research support; *Bulletin of the Hospital for Joint Disease*: editorial or governing board; *Clinical Orthopaedics and Related Research*: editorial or governing board; DJ Orthopaedics: paid consultant; Ferring Pharmaceuticals: research support; Force Therapeutics: stock or stock options; Hip Society: board or committee member; *JBJS Reviews*: editorial or governing board; *Journal of Arthroplasty*: editorial or governing board; *Journal of Bone and Joint Surgery–American*: editorial or governing board; *Journal of the American Academy of Orthopaedic Surgeons*: editorial or governing board; Knee Society: board or committee member; MCS ActiveCare: paid consultant; stock or stock options; Medtronic: paid consultant; Muve Health: paid consultant; stock or stock options; Orthofix, Inc: research support; Orthosensor: research support; Pacira: paid consultant, research support; URX Mobile: stock or stock options; Vericel: research support; Wellbe: stock or stock options.

REFERENCES

1. Mihalko WM, Bergin PF, Kelly FB. Obesity, orthopaedics, and outcomes. J Am Acad Orthop Surg 2014;22(11):683–90.
2. Ogden CL, Carroll MD, Fryar CD, et al. Prevalence of obesity among adults and youth: United States, 2011-2014. NCHS Data Brief 2015;(219):1–8.
3. Heymsfield SB, Wadden TA. Mechanisms, pathophysiology, and management of obesity. N Engl J Med 2017;376(3):254–66.
4. Haynes J, Nam D, Barrack RL. Obesity in total hip arthroplasty: does it make a difference? Bone Joint J 2017;99-B(1 Supple A):31–6.
5. World Health Organization. Obesity: preventing and managing the global epidemic. WHO Technical Report Series; 2000. p. 894.
6. Koonce RC, Bravman JT. Obesity and osteoarthritis: more than just wear and tear. J Am Acad Orthop Surg 2013;21(3):161–9.
7. Recnik G, Kralj-Iglič V, Iglič A, et al. The role of obesity, biomechanical constitution of the pelvis and contact joint stress in progression of hip osteoarthritis. Osteoarthr Cartil 2009;17(7):879–82.
8. Bourne R, Mukhi S, Zhu N, et al. Role of obesity on the risk for total hip or knee arthroplasty. Clin Orthop Relat Res 2007;465:185–8.
9. Losina E, Walensky RP, Reichmann WM, et al. Impact of obesity and knee osteoarthritis on morbidity and mortality in older Americans. Ann Intern Med 2011;154(4):217–26.
10. Martin JR, Jennings JM, Dennis DA. Morbid obesity and total knee arthroplasty: a growing problem. J Am Acad Orthop Surg 2017;25(3):188–94.

11. Watts CD, Houdek MT, Wagner ER, et al. Insulin dependence increases the risk of failure after total knee arthroplasty in morbidly obese patients. J Arthroplasty 2016;31(1):256–9.

12. Watts CD, Martin JR, Houdek MT, et al. Prior bariatric surgery may decrease the rate of reoperation and revision following total hip arthroplasty. Bone Joint J 2016;98-B(9):1180–4.

13. Smith TO, Aboelmagd T, Hing CB, et al. Does bariatric surgery prior to total hip or knee arthroplasty reduce post-operative complications and improve clinical outcomes for obese patients? Systematic review and meta-analysis. Bone Joint J 2016;98-B(9):1160–6.

14. Peterson LA, Cheskin LJ, Furtado M, et al. Malnutrition in bariatric surgery candidates: multiple micronutrient deficiencies prior to surgery. Obes Surg 2016;26(4):833–8.

15. Gage MJ, Schwarzkopf R, Abrouk M, et al. Impact of metabolic syndrome on perioperative complication rates after total joint arthroplasty surgery. J Arthroplasty 2014;29(9):1842–5.

16. Schwarzkopf R, Thompson SL, Adwar SJ, et al. Postoperative complication rates in the "super-obese" hip and knee arthroplasty population. J Arthroplasty 2012;27(3):397–401.

17. Dowsey MM, Choong PFM. Obese diabetic patients are at substantial risk for deep infection after primary TKA. Clin Orthop Relat Res 2009;467(6): 1577–81.

18. Tayton ER, Frampton C, Hooper GJ, et al. The impact of patient and surgical factors on the rate of infection after primary total knee arthroplasty: an analysis of 64 566 joints from the New Zealand Joint Registry. Bone Joint J 2016;98-B(3):334–40.

19. Namba RS, Inacio MCS, Paxton EW. Risk factors associated with deep surgical site infections after primary total knee arthroplasty: an analysis of 56,216 knees. J Bone Joint Surg Am 2013;95(9): 775–82.

20. Maoz G, Phillips M, Bosco J, et al. The Otto Aufranc Award: modifiable versus nonmodifiable risk factors for infection after hip arthroplasty. Clin Orthop Relat Res 2014;473(2):1–7.

21. Watts CD, Wagner ER, Houdek MT, et al. Morbid obesity: a significant risk factor for failure of two-stage revision total knee arthroplasty for infection. J Bone Joint Surg Am 2014;96(18):e154.

22. Davis AM, Wood AM, Keenan ACM, et al. Does body mass index affect clinical outcome post-operatively and at five years after primary unilateral total hip replacement performed for osteoarthritis? A multivariate analysis of prospective data. J Bone Joint Surg Br 2011;93(9):1178–82.

23. Elkins JM, Daniel M, Pedersen DR, et al. Morbid obesity may increase dislocation in total hip patients: a biomechanical analysis. Clin Orthop Relat Res 2013;471(3):971–80.

24. Huffman KD, Sanford BA, Zucker-Levin AR, et al. Increased hip abduction in high body mass index subjects during sit-to-stand. Gait Posture 2015; 41(2):640–5.

25. Kerkhoffs GMMJ, Servien E, Dunn W, et al. The influence of obesity on the complication rate and outcome of total knee arthroplasty. J Bone Joint Surg Am 2012;94(20):1839–44.

26. Abdel MP, Bonadurer GF, Jennings MT, et al. Increased aseptic tibial failures in patients with a BMI ≥35 and well-aligned total knee arthroplasties. J Arthroplasty 2015;30(12):2181–4.

27. Vazquez-Vela Johnson G, Worland RL, Keenan J, et al. Patient demographics as a predictor of the ten-year survival rate in primary total knee replacement. J Bone Joint Surg Br 2003;85(1):52–6.

28. Mulhall KJ, Ghomrawi HM, Mihalko W, et al. Adverse effects of increased body mass index and weight on survivorship of total knee arthroplasty and subsequent outcomes of revision TKA. J Knee Surg 2007;20(3):199–204.

29. Electricwala AJ, Narkbunnam R, Huddleston JI, et al. Obesity is associated with early total hip revision for aseptic loosening. J Arthroplasty 2016;31(9 Suppl):217–20.

30. Haverkamp D, Klinkenbijl MN, Somford MP, et al. Obesity in total hip arthroplasty–does it really matter? A meta-analysis. Acta Orthop 2011;82(4): 417–22.

31. Issa K, Harwin SF, Malkani AL, et al. Bariatric Orthopaedics: total hip arthroplasty in super-obese patients (those with a BMI of ≥50 kg/m2). J Bone Joint Surg Am 2016;98(3):180–5.

32. Friedman RJ, Hess S, Berkowitz SD, et al. Complication rates after hip or knee arthroplasty in morbidly obese patients. Clin Orthop Relat Res 2013;471(10):3358–66.

33. D'Apuzzo MR, Novicoff WM, Browne JA. The John Insall Award: morbid obesity independently impacts complications, mortality, and resource use after TKA. Clin Orthop Relat Res 2015;473(1):57–63.

34. Naziri Q, Issa K, Malkani AL, et al. Bariatric orthopaedics: total knee arthroplasty in super-obese patients (BMI > 50 kg/m2). Survivorship and complications. Clin Orthop Relat Res 2013; 471(11):3523–30.

35. Chee YH, Teoh KH, Sabnis BM, et al. Total hip replacement in morbidly obese patients with osteoarthritis: results of a prospectively matched study. J Bone Joint Surg Br 2010;92(8):1066–71.

The Role of Bariatric Surgery in the Obese Total Joint Arthroplasty Patient

Jessica M. Hooper, MD[a], Ajit J. Deshmukh, MD[b],
Ran Schwarzkopf, MD, MSc[c],*

KEYWORDS

• Bariatric surgery • Arthroplasty • Risk modification • Outcomes • Complications • Readmissions

---

KEY POINTS

- Morbid obesity (BMI > 40 kg/m^2) greatly increases the risk profile associated with total joint arthroplasty, and bariatric surgery is proven means of weight loss and comorbidity reduction in this high-risk patient population.
- Obesity changes the mechanical axis and loading patterns in the lower extremity, which may affect implant loading, and therefore wear profiles, in this patient population.
- Weight loss after bariatric surgery may reduce pain and disability associated with osteoarthritis, and the radiographic appearance of disease.
- Current data on efficacy of bariatric surgery in reducing risks associated with TJA in the morbidly obese patient population are mixed and are based exclusively on retrospective studies.
- Bariatric surgery may lead to substantial cost savings in the arthroplasty population, both related to health care resource utilization and to reduced incidence of adverse events after TJA.

INTRODUCTION

Obesity, defined as a body mass index (BMI) greater than 30 kg/m^2, contributes to many chronic medical conditions, such as obstructive sleep apnea, hypertension, hyperlipidemia, diabetes mellitus, and cardiovascular disease,[1] and its prevalence in American adults is steadily increasing.[2,3] Obese adults are more likely to be malnourished and have other metabolic derangements than their nonobese peers, which

contribute to a state of poor overall health.[1,4–11] Obesity has been identified as an independent risk factor for the development of osteoarthritis; excess body weight increases loads at the hips and knees, accelerating cartilage degeneration.[12,13] The excess adipose tissue in obese patients acts like an endocrine organ, generating and releasing proinflammatory mediators that may further contribute to articular cartilage damage.[14–16] Obese patients are often younger when they are considered for total joint

---

Disclosure Statement: Dr J.M. Hooper reports no grants, personal fees, royalties, or payments related to this submitted work. Dr A.J. Deshmukh reports no grants, personal fees, royalties, or payments related to this submitted work. Dr R. Schwarzkopf reports grants and personal fees from Smith and Nephew, and personal fees from Intellijoint, neither of which are related to the submitted work.

[a] Department of Orthopaedic Surgery, New York University Langone Orthopaedic Hospital, 301 East 17th Street, New York, NY 10003, USA; [b] Department of Adult Reconstruction, New York University Langone Orthopaedic Hospital, 301 East 17th Street, New York, NY 10003, USA; [c] Adult Reconstructive Surgery, Department of Adult Reconstruction, New York University Langone Orthopaedic Hospital, 301 East 17th Street, Suite 1402, New York, NY 10003, USA

* Corresponding author.
E-mail address: ran.schwarzkopf@nyumc.org

Orthop Clin N Am 49 (2018) 297–306
https://doi.org/10.1016/j.ocl.2018.02.003

arthroplasty (TJA), and are at increased risk for perioperative complications and readmissions.[17–22] To help reduce the risk of complications, bariatric surgery is often recommended for morbidly obese patients being considered for TJA.

Bariatric surgery has proven to be a more effective means of weight loss than nonsurgical interventions in the morbidly obese patient population (BMI > 40 kg/m²), and can help induce partial or complete remission of obesity-related comorbidities, such as type 2 diabetes mellitus, hypertension, and dyslipidemia.[5] This article reviews the effects of obesity on arthroplasty surgery outcomes, metabolic changes associated with bariatric surgery, the role of bariatric surgery as a risk-modification tool, specific considerations for perioperative care of the bariatric surgery patient undergoing TJA, and the impact of these interventions on perioperative outcomes.

EFFECTS OF OBESITY ON ARTHROPLASTY OUTCOMES

Because of increased body weight and associated changes in body habitus, obese patients often modify their gait to decrease lower extremity joint loading. The knee is consistently subjected to greater loads than the hip.[23] A recent meta-analysis found that obese patients have a lower walking velocity, an increased toe-out angle, and a greater absolute adduction moment compared with normal-weight individuals.[24] Obese individuals compensate for the increased abduction moment at the hip by widening their stance and abducting the hips, especially during high-demand tasks, such as sit-to-stand.[25] At the knee, it is hypothesized that elevated body weight and an increased adduction moment loads the articular cartilage in the medial compartment beyond its yield point, causing irreversible changes. After an obese patient undergoes total knee arthroplasty (TKA), the bearing surfaces bear the excess load, and the adduction moment persists.[26] Obese patients are at increased risk of accelerated bearing surface wear, implant loosening, and early prosthesis failure compared with normal-weight patients who undergo TKA and total hip arthroplasty (THA).[13,18–20,27]

In addition to mechanical issues related to implant loading, TJA is more technically difficult in obese patients. Multiple studies have demonstrated a higher number of technical errors occurring in obese patients.[20,30] The 2013

American Association of Hip and Knee Surgeons expert workgroup on obesity in arthroplasty patients concluded that obese patients are at increased risk of surgical site infections, periprosthetic joint infections, respiratory complications, thromboembolic events, need for revision surgery, component malposition, and prosthetic loosening.[21] Obese patients are also more likely to have an increased length of stay and elevated total cost associated with their TJA procedure.[21] The overall rate of complications after TJA increases from 5% to 22%, and the rate of periprosthetic joint infection increases from 0.37% to 4.66% in morbidly obese patients.[22,31] Perioperative risk has also been shown to increase with higher BMIs; Schwarzkopf and colleagues[18] demonstrated that each incremental 5-unit increase in BMI higher than 45 kg/m² was associated with a statistically significant increased risk of in-hospital complications (odds ratio [OR], 1.69), postoperative outpatient complications (OR, 2.71), and readmissions (OR, 2). The official recommendation of the American Association of Hip and Knee Surgeons workgroup was for weight loss before proceeding with TJA in the morbidly obese population.

Given the increasing prevalence of obesity in the TJA patient population, bariatric surgery is often offered to morbidly obese patients with end-stage arthropathy as a legitimate means for weight loss, overall health improvement, and reducing perioperative arthroplasty risks.

BARIATRIC SURGICAL OPTIONS

In the general population, bariatric surgery is offered to patients with BMI greater than 40 or to patients with BMI greater than 35 and the presence of obesity-related comorbidities, because higher grades of obesity are associated with excess mortality from cardiovascular disease and diabetes.[3,32] Although evidence has shown that bariatric surgery effectively reduces weight and decreases the burden of obesity-related comorbidities, there is insufficient evidence to support offering bariatric surgery to nonobese patients specifically for glycemic control or cardiac disease risk reduction.[32] Because of the well-demonstrated risk increase associated with BMI greater than 40 in patients undergoing TJA, orthopedic surgeons often refer obese patients indicated for TJA for consultation with bariatric surgeons.

Bariatric surgical procedures are defined as restrictive (laparoscopic adjustable gastric banding [LAGB], laparoscopic sleeve gastrectomy [LSG]), malabsorptive, or combined (laparoscopic Roux-en-Y gastric bypass [LRYGB], laparoscopic biliopancreatic diversion [BPD], BPD with duodenal switch [BPD/DS]), based on the surgical methods used to effect weight loss (Table 1).[32] Procedure choice is based on individualized goals of therapy, surgeon and institutional expertise, patient preferences, and risk stratification. Although many patients experience high percentage excess weight loss (% EWL) following malabsorptive and combined procedures, the risk of associated nutritional derangements and vitamin and mineral deficiencies is also high, because of the reduced surface area for nutrient absorption in the bypassed small intestine.[32]

With improvements in bariatric surgical technique, associated mortality rates after bariatric surgery have decreased.[33,34] A recent meta-analysis by Chang and colleagues[33] found that estimated mortality rates in current studies are

Table 1
Types of bariatric surgery

Procedure	Abbreviation	Procedure Type	Description
Laparoscopic adjustable gastric banding	LAGB	Restrictive	Placement of silicone band around the proximal stomach; restricts solid food intake Band is adjustable; controlled by injection/withdrawal of saline into band through subcutaneous access port
Laparoscopic sleeve gastrectomy	LSG	Restrictive	Gastric division in a vertical fashion, retaining only the lesser curvature of the stomach and the native pylorus; restricts solid food intake
Laparoscopic Roux-en-Y gastric bypass	LRYGB	Combined	Creation of a vertically oriented proximal gastric pouch; restricts solid food intake Jejunum is divided, creating a 75- to 150-cm Roux limb, which is then used to create a jejunojejunostomy; limits absorption of calories and nutrients
Laparoscopic biliopancreatic diversion	BPD	Combined	Distal subtotal gastrectomy; restricts solid food intake Roux-en-Y anastomosis created 50–110 cm proximal to the ileocecal valve, and distal 250 cm of small intestine is anastomosed to the gastric pouch with a 2- to 3-cm stoma; limits absorption of calories and nutrients
Laparoscopic biliopancreatic diversion with duodenal switch	BPD/DS	Combined	Subtotal gastrectomy, retaining narrow lesser curvature tube of stomach; restricts solid food intake, reduces incidence of marginal ulcers Roux-en-Y anastomosis created 50–110 cm proximal to the ileocecal valve, and distal 250 cm of small intestine is anastomosed to the gastric pouch with a 2- to 3-cm stoma; limits absorption of calories and nutrients

Data from Schauer PR, Schirmer B. The surgical management of obesity. In: Brunicardi FC, Andersen DK, Billiar TR, et al, editors. Schwartz's principles of surgery. 10th edition. New York: McGraw-Hill Education; 2015.

lower than what has been reported in previous meta-analyses: perioperative mortality rate ranges from 0.08% to 0.22%, and postoperative mortality ranges from 0.31% to 0.33%. Although the general safety profile and expected outcomes of each procedure can be estimated, it is difficult to predict an individual's response to bariatric surgery in terms of %EWL and treatment of associated comorbidities over time. Among the different surgical options, LAGB is associated with lower mortality and complication rates, lower weight loss, and higher reoperation rate.[33] LSG is more effective in achieving weight loss than LAGB, and is comparable with LRYGB with respect to maintained weight loss at 5 years.[33] A meta-analysis by Zhang and colleagues[34] reviewing postoperative metabolic effects of bariatric procedures found that LRYGB and LSG have an equivalent effect on hypertension and dyslipidemia, but LRYGB facilitated superior control of type 2 diabetes mellitus. Overall, BPD/DS effects the most BMI loss among all procedures, but the procedures with a malabsorptive component, such as BPD/DS, have higher mortality and complication rates.[33] Therefore, it seems that procedures associated with greater weight loss also carry increased risk of complications and post-procedure sequelae, such as malnutrition and vitamin deficiencies, which should not be ignored in this patient population, given the implications for wound healing and infectious complications.

EFFECT OF BARIATRIC SURGERY ON OSTEOARTHRITIS

In addition to the multiple metabolic consequences of bariatric surgery, several studies have also assessed the effect of bariatric surgery on joint pain, function, and progression of osteoarthritis in morbidly obese patients.[35,36] A greater improvement is consistently seen in knee osteoarthritis symptoms compared with hip symptoms in obese patients following substantial weight loss, likely because the knee bears greater loads in standing and gait.[23,37] In the knee, the effect of weight loss on improvements in patient function and knee symptoms is usually dose-dependent; patients who lose more weight experience greater alleviation of symptoms.[13] In their prospective review patients with osteoarthritis and mean BMI of 43 kg/m² who underwent LAGB, Abu-Abeid and co-workers[38] found that within 3 months of surgery, radiographic improvement of knee osteoarthritis was seen, and clinically relevant improvement in pain and function (American Knee Society

Scores). Mean BMI decreased to 37 kg/m². Korenkov and colleagues[4] reported on 145 obese patients (mean BMI, 49 kg/m²) with knee osteoarthritis who underwent LAGB. In mid and long term follow up (3–8 years), there was a statistically significant decrease in percentage of patients complaining of knee pain (47% to 38%; $P<.001$), and in the intensity of reported knee pain (3–1, numeric rating scale; $P<.001$).

Hooper and colleagues[39] conducted a study looking at the effect of weight loss on specific musculoskeletal conditions in obese patients following RYGB. With a decrease in mean BMI from 51 to 36 kg/m² over 6 to 12 months after surgery, there was a significant improvement in symptoms at the knee and foot, although there was minimal improvement in hip pain and trochanteric bursal pain.[39] In this study, improvement was quantified by patient-reported pain and responses to standardized questionnaires (Short Form-36 and Western Ontario and McMaster Universities Osteoarthritis Index [WOMAC]), and there was no correlation of reported symptoms with radiographic evidence of osteoarthritis. Biomechanical studies of gait changes in obese subjects who undergo bariatric surgery have demonstrated significant decreases in step width in the frontal plane,[40,41] which also reduces the adduction moment at the knee and the flexion angle at the hip.

Most published evidence demonstrates that bariatric surgery reduces hip and knee pain and stiffness, and improves range of motion in obese patients with osteoarthritis.[21,36] One study, a retrospective report of 15 obese patients (mean BMI, 52 kg/m²) with osteoarthritis who underwent bariatric surgery, found that patients who had bariatric surgery and went on to TJA had a greater change in BMI than those who did not eventually go on to TJA ($P = .049$).[42] The authors speculated that greater weight loss may have accelerated osteoarthritis progression in their cohort because of increased physical activity following weight loss. Although this explanation for this specific patient cohort is plausible, the expanding body of literature on physical activity in obese patients after bariatric surgery indicates that these patients have a similar activity level to the general population,[43] and a significant change in activity level is not anticipated after bariatric surgery.[44] Trofa and colleagues[42] did not compare the prebariatric surgery radiographic and clinical severity of osteoarthritis between patients who went on to TJA and those who did not. The findings of Trofa and colleagues[42] can best be interpreted as obese patients with osteoarthritis who increase their activity level significantly after bariatric surgery are more likely to go on to TJA, independent of the amount of weight loss.

EFFECT OF BARIATRIC SURGERY ON ARTHROPLASTY OUTCOMES

In theory, bariatric surgery leads to weight loss and reduction of obesity-related comorbidities, both of which are known to increase the risk of adverse events after TJA.[18,31,45] This is a topic of much scholarly interest, because the available data on the actual effect of bariatric surgery on arthroplasty outcomes are based on retrospective case control studies, and have presented mixed results.

In one of the largest studies to date, Werner and colleagues[46] compared 11,294 morbidly obese patients who underwent TKA with 219 morbidly obese patients who had bariatric surgery. Their results demonstrated that the patients who underwent bariatric surgery first had half the rate of major complications (OR, $P = .001$), and 40% fewer minor complications (OR .61, $P = .01$). Kulkarni and colleagues[47] identified 143 obese patients who underwent both bariatric surgery and TJA. The 53 patients who received bariatric surgery first had a 3.5 times lower wound infection rate and 7 times lower readmission rate than the 90 patients who had TJA before bariatric surgery.

Despite these encouraging findings, other studies have not demonstrated a reduction in complications.[48] Severson and colleagues[48] found that obese patients who underwent TJA greater than 2 years after bariatric surgery had shorter operative times and anesthesia times, but no significant difference in length of hospital stay or 90-day complication rates compared with patients who underwent TJA less than 2 years after bariatric surgery. Using Kaiser Permanente data, Inacio and colleagues[49] found that bariatric surgery before TJA did not reduce the frequency of complications, readmissions, deep surgical site infections, or revision following TJA. A matched cohort study conducted by Martin and colleagues[50] found that obese patients who underwent bariatric surgery before TKA had a higher risk of, and worse survival free of, TKA reoperation compared with patients who had not undergone bariatric surgery, regardless of BMI. The mean BMI in the bariatric surgery cohort dropped to 37.3 kg/m^2 from 51.1 kg/m^2 before TKA. The results of this study in particular suggest that the metabolic consequences of bariatric surgery cannot be ignored, because

weight loss after bariatric surgery did not improve the risk profile associated with TJA.

TIMING OF SURGERY

When considering bariatric surgery before TJA specifically for risk reduction, the optimal timing for each procedure is not obvious. Most weight loss after bariatric surgery occurs 1 to 2 years after the procedure, and is maintained thereafter in most patients.[51] Theoretically, increasing the time from bariatric surgery to elective TJA would increase the metabolic and musculoskeletal benefits of bariatric surgery, and may obviate arthroplasty altogether in patients with severe pain without end-stage disease.

It is well documented that undergoing TJA does not result in substantial weight loss for patients.[52,53] The only clinically significant predictor of weight loss after TJA was age; older patients were more likely to lose weight after surgery than younger patients.[53] It is also well known that many morbidly obese patients have negative attitudes toward physical activity,[43] which suggests that a significant increase in physical activity after surgery should not be expected, because there is a strong psychological component to a patient's ability and willingness to participate in physical activity. Even for a willing obese patient, participation in regular exercise without dietary modifications does not lead to significant weight loss.[53,54] Despite the best intentions, obese patients undergoing TJA will likely remain at significantly increased risk of complications related to their weight and associated medical comorbidities.

No studies have yet been able to make a definitive recommendation on the optimal timing for TJA following bariatric surgery. There are several potential explanations for this ambiguity. First, the time course of any individual patient's response to bariatric surgery in unpredictable and multifactorial. Golomb and colleagues[5] found that the %EWL and rates of partial and complete remission of type 2 diabetes mellitus were significantly lower with increased time from LSG. Additionally, the type of bariatric surgery, restrictive or malabsorptive, also affects the observed postoperative weight loss and metabolic changes. Previous studies have shown that the metabolic benefits of LRYGB are apparent before substantial weight loss occurs, whereas weight loss occurs before metabolic changes after restrictive procedures, such as LSG.[6,55] Comparing restrictive procedures and malabsorptive procedures, Shoar and Saber[7] found that LRYGB produced greater long-term weight loss than LSG, although no difference was noted in the rate of reduction of comorbidities. The potential nutritional deficiencies associated with bariatric surgeries do not develop immediately.[32] In particular, patients who undergo malabsorptive surgery are at increased risk for nutritional deficiencies that may have deleterious effects on bone density, which may increase the risk of late adverse events.[56,57]

Further complicating the picture, there have been no studies published looking at bariatric surgery done specifically for risk reduction before TJA. The available data include patients who may have had bariatric surgery several years before developing end-stage osteoarthritis and undergoing TJA and have thus had ample time for weight loss and metabolic changes to equilibrate. There are also ethical concerns associated with having obese, and likely debilitated, patients with end-stage osteoarthritis wait years after bariatric surgery to undergo joint replacement. Published evidence suggests that waiting more than 6 months for total hip arthroplasty leads to poorer physical function and poorer function after surgery.[58] Prospective or randomized trials are needed to better evaluate the ideal timing for TJA after bariatric surgery.

THE ETHICS OF PERIOPERATIVE RISK MODIFICATION

TJA is one of the most commonly performed elective surgeries in the United States, and part of its enormous popularity is related to the low rates of serious complications. However, all arthroplasty surgeons know that serious complications, either medical or orthopedic, impose major morbidity on patients expecting a quick recovery. The principles of risk modification cannot be ignored; even staunch advocates of patient autonomy can appreciate that, for many patients, an attempt to decrease the modifiable risks for complications in elective TJA would likely be beneficial for surgeons and patients. Morbid obesity and diabetes mellitus are two patient factors strongly associated with complications related to TJA.[13,21,59]

Bariatric surgery is an aggressive risk modification tool when compared with other interventions, such as smoking cessation counseling, improved glycemic control, or nonsurgical weight loss, and it should not be considered a benign procedure. The overall complication rate ranges from 10% to 17%, and data from randomized controlled trials have demonstrated a lower rate of complications with sleeve gastrectomy (13%) and adjustable gastric banding (13%), compared with LRYGB (21%).[33] Because bariatric surgery causes weight loss and often resolution of comorbidities, it may improve the risk profile for morbidly obese patients indicated for TJA.

Detractors of aggressive interventional risk modification argue that the risks associated with delaying TJA are not worth the potential benefits of bariatric surgery. In addition to worsening quality of life and loss of function, published data also suggest that delaying TJA may worsen overall postoperative outcomes.[45] Patients with severe arthropathy who delay TJA may also become debilitated to the point of being unable to work, increasing personal and societal costs.[58] Although the optimal time to operate is not clearly defined, and is likely variable among patients, delaying TJA in the name of risk modification will become increasingly necessary because of fiscal and societal pressures on the health care system as a whole.[59] Bariatric surgery before TJA is certainly not necessary for all obese patients, but it is a conversation worth having with morbidly obese patients with metabolic syndrome being considered for TJA. Physician and patient collaboration using a shared decision-making model helps patients make informed choices about their health care, such as choosing to accept the increased risk of complications if risk-modifying interventions, such as bariatric surgery, are waived in favor of undergoing TJA sooner or pursuing nonsurgical weight loss. Incorporating patient goals and preferences into the decision-making process leads to increased satisfaction, compliance, and outcomes.[60] Ideally, the arthroplasty surgeon, the bariatric surgeon, and the patient should discuss goals of care together.

ECONOMIC CONSIDERATIONS

Patients who are overweight or obese impose a significant economic burden on society. In addition to potential for indirect costs related to lost work hours because of arthritis-related disability, direct health care costs incurred by obese patients with arthritis are more than triple the cost compared with normal-weight patients with arthritis.[61] Given that the costs to patients and society from arthritis in the obese patient population are so high, it is reasonable to consider that the upfront costs of TJA may be worth later savings.

Unfortunately, the significantly increased risk of intraoperative and postoperative complications associated with TJA in this patient population may not justify the potential cost savings.[13,18–22,27,30] A study by Culler and colleagues[62] looking at beneficiaries within the Medicare Provider Analysis Review file demonstrated that any adverse event significantly increased mean hospital cost by $3429, and increased length of stay by 1 day. A subsequent study was conducted by the same group assessing the economic implications of adverse events in the TJA population within the Center for Medicare and Medicaid Services' Comprehensive Joint Replacement Bundled Payment Initiative.[63] Considering only major adverse events, defined as in-hospital death, acute myocardial infarction, pneumonia, sepsis/septic shock, surgical bleeding, pulmonary embolism, periprosthetic joint infection, and mechanical complications, the authors found that the mean incremental cost to the hospital was $12,007 per patient if any of these adverse events occurred.[63] Within the framework of bundled payment for arthroplasty cases, the authors propose that all possible quality improvement interventions should be undertaken to reduce the risk of adverse events, and therefore reduce hospital costs. Keeping costs low whenever possible allows physicians and hospitals to better absorb costs associated with unanticipated adverse events in patients believed to be at low risk. This evidence suggests that there are potential health care savings to be realized if weight loss is addressed in morbidly obese patients before TJA.[64]

The economics of bariatric surgery have been well published. It is an expensive intervention; costs accumulate because of preoperative referrals and testing, inpatient and surgical costs, and postoperative costs related to short- and long-term complications.[65] It is necessary to weigh the costs associated with an obese patient undergoing bariatric surgery against the anticipated expenditures for the management of obesity-related health care problems (the cost of not having bariatric surgery).

Lewis and colleagues[66] conducted a study comparing costs associated with LAGB and LRYGB. They demonstrated that the trend of total health care and prescription drug costs flattened 3 years after both types of bariatric surgery, indicating that bariatric surgery has the potential to produce long-term cost savings in this patient population. LAGB was associated with lower costs and fewer emergency department visits in the early postoperative period, because of lower risk of adverse events, but by 3 years after surgery, LRYGB resulted in significantly lower total and prescription drug costs. Just as gastric bypass has been demonstrated to have greater success with weight loss and comorbidity reduction,[5,34] it also translates into greater long-term health care savings. As the popularity of the LSG increases, further study is needed to determine how it compares with LRGYB from an economic perspective.

Published evidence indicates that costs associated with the management of arthritis in the obese patient population far exceed costs for normal-weight patients.[61] Additionally, obesity and associated comorbidities increase the likelihood of complications following TJA, and complications increase the health care costs associated with the surgical encounter. Bariatric surgery can lead to resolution of obesity and related comorbidities and has been shown to decrease health care expenditures. Considering bariatric surgery for patients with end-stage arthropathy through the lens of risk reduction for TJA, it seems reasonable to extrapolate the projected long-term savings to this patient population.

McLawhorn and coworkers[67] conducted a computer-based evaluation using a Markov model to compare cost utility of bariatric surgery in patients with morbid obesity and end-stage knee arthropathy. Their results indicate that morbidly obese patients who underwent bariatric surgery 2 years before TKA had higher quality-adjusted life years than morbidly obese patients who received TKA alone. The incremental cost-effectiveness ratio between these two groups was $13,910 per quality-adjusted life year, which indicates that use of bariatric surgery for risk reduction before TKA may be cost-effective from a societal perspective. To our knowledge, there has not yet been a study using clinical data that would support these results, and it remains to be seen if these numbers hold up for all types of bariatric surgery, with their varying complication and weight loss rates.

The data on efficacy of bariatric surgery for improvement of arthroplasty outcomes are mixed,[13] which can perhaps be attributed to the fact that the optimal timing for arthroplasty after bariatric surgery is not yet well-defined. The model constructed by McLawhorn and coworkers[67] supposes a 2-year waiting period from bariatric surgery to TJA, which may not be practical for all patients. Additional clinical studies are needed to validate this model and help surgeons and policy-makers find the "sweet spot" - the optimal timing to maximize weight loss and metabolic benefit after bariatric surgery, maximize economic benefit, and reduce the risks associated with TJA.

SUMMARY

Obesity and its comorbidities place patients at increased risk for perioperative complications following TJA, especially when BMI exceeds 40 kg/m². Bariatric surgery has proven to be a successful intervention for weight loss and co-morbidity reduction and is associated with a low mortality rate. As the indications for bariatric surgery and TJA expand, understanding how the two procedures can affect each other becomes increasingly important. Based on the current evidence, the ideal patient for whom preoperative bariatric surgery is reasonably considered for risk reduction before TJA has BMI greater than 40 kg/m², at least one obesity-related medical problem, and end-stage arthropathy with symptoms unlikely to resolve with weight loss. Morbidly obese patients should be explicitly made aware that their risk of perioperative complications is greatly increased by their obesity, and that they should not expect major increases in their activity level leading to weight loss after TJA. Further study is needed to better evaluate the effect of bariatric surgery on arthroplasty outcomes and determine the optimal timing for both surgical procedures. On an individual level, the decision to proceed with bariatric surgery before TJA should be made by the patient, the orthopedic surgeon, and the bariatric surgeon together, and should be based on realistic expectations. On a population level, indicating patients for bariatric surgery before TJA may substantially reduce costs in this patient population. Surgeons, administrators, and policy-makers should consider all of these factors when developing institutional protocols for the management of morbidly obese patients with end-stage osteoarthritis.

REFERENCES

1. Guh DP, Zhang W, Bansback N, et al. The incidence of co-morbidities related to obesity and overweight: a systematic review and meta-analysis. BMC Public Health 2009;9(1):88.
2. Nguyen DM, El-Serag HB. The epidemiology of obesity. Gastroenterol Clin North Am 2010;39(1): 1–7.
3. Flegal KM, Carroll MD, Ogden CL, et al. Prevalence and trends in obesity among US adults, 1999–2008. JAMA 2010;303(3):235–41.
4. Korenkov M, Shah S, Sauerland S, et al. Impact of laparoscopic adjustable gastric banding on obesity co-morbidities in the medium-and long-term. Obes Surg 2007;17(5):679–83.
5. Golomb I, Ben David M, Glass A, et al. Long-term metabolic effects of laparoscopic sleeve gastrectomy. JAMA Surg 2015;150(11):1051–7.
6. Thaler JP, Cummings DE. Hormonal and metabolic mechanisms of diabetes remission after gastrointestinal surgery. Endocrinology 2009; 150(6):2518–25.
7. Shoar S, Saber AA. Long-term and midterm outcomes of laparoscopic sleeve gastrectomy versus Roux-en-Y gastric bypass: a systematic review and meta-analysis of comparative studies. Surg Obes Relat Dis 2017;13(2):170–80.
8. Haslam DW, James WP. Obesity. Lancet 2005; 366(9492):1197–209.
9. Hubert HB, Feinleb M, McNamara PM, et al. Obesity as an independent risk factor for cardiovascular disease: a 26-year follow-up of participants in the Framingham Heart Study. Circulation 1983; 67(5):968–77.
10. Ejerblad E, Fored CM, Lindblad P, et al. Obesity and risk for chronic renal failure. J Am Soc Nephrol 2006;17(6):1695–702.
11. Myles TD, Gooch J, Santolaya J. Obesity as an independent risk factor for infectious morbidity in patients who undergo cesarean delivery. Obstet Gynecol 2002;100(5, pt 1):959–64.
12. Blagojevic M, Jinks C, Jeffery A, et al. Risk factors for onset of osteoarthritis of the knee in older adults: a systematic review and meta-analysis. Osteoarthritis Cartilage 2010;18(1):24–33.
13. Springer BD, Carter JT, McLawhorn AS, et al. Obesity and the role of bariatric surgery in the surgical management of osteoarthritis of the hip and knee: a review of the literature. Surg Obes Relat Dis 2017;13(1):111–8.
14. Abramson SB, Attur M. Developments in the scientific understanding of osteoarthritis. Arthritis Res Ther 2009;11(3):227.
15. Griffin TM, Guilak F. Why is obesity associated with osteoarthritis? Insights from mouse models of obesity. Biorheology 2008;45(3–4):387–98.
16. Messier SP. Obesity and osteoarthritis: disease genesis and nonpharmacologic weight management. Rheum Dis Clin North Am 2008;34(3): 713–29.
17. Davis AM, Wood AM, Keenan ACM, et al. Does body mass index affect clinical outcome postoperatively and at five years after primary unilateral total hip replacement performed for osteoarthritis? J Bone Joint Surg Br 2011;93(9):1178–82.

18. Schwarzkopf R, Thompson SL, Adwar SJ, et al. Postoperative complication rates in the "super-obese" hip and knee arthroplasty population. J Arthroplasty 2012;27(3):397–401.

19. Abdel MP, Bonadurer GF, Jennings MT, et al. Increased aseptic tibial failures in patients with a BMI ≥35 and well-aligned total knee arthroplasties. J Arthroplasty 2015;30(12):2181–4.

20. Kerkhoffs GMMJ, Servien E, Dunn W, et al. The influence of obesity on the complication rate and outcome of total knee arthroplasty: a meta-analysis and systematic literature review. J Bone Joint Surg Am 2012;94(20):1839–44.

21. Workgroup of the American Association of Hip and Knee Surgeons Evidence Based Committee. Obesity and total joint arthroplasty. J Arthroplasty 2013;28(5):714–21.

22. Jämsen E, Nevalainen P, Eskelinen A, et al. Obesity, diabetes, and preoperative hyperglycemia as predictors of periprosthetic joint infection: a single-center analysis of 7181 primary hip and knee replacements for osteoarthritis. J Bone Joint Surg Am 2012;94(14):e101.

23. Taylor WR, Heller MO, Bergmann G, et al. Tibio-femoral loading during human gait and stair climbing. J Orthop Res 2004;22(3):625–32.

24. Runhaar J, Koes BW, Clockaerts S, et al. A systematic review on changed biomechanics of lower extremities in obese individuals: a possible role in development of osteoarthritis. Obes Rev 2011;12(12):1071–82.

25. Huffman KD, Sanford BA, Zucker-Levin AR, et al. Increased hip abduction in high body mass index subjects during sit-to-stand. Gait Posture 2015; 41(2):640–5.

26. Orishimo KF, Kremenic IJ, Deshmukh AJ, et al. Does total knee arthroplasty change frontal plane knee biomechanics during gait? Clin Orthop Relat Res 2012;470(4):1171–6.

27. Vazquez-Vela Johnson G, Worland RL, Keenan J, et al. Patient demographics as a predictor of the ten-year survival rate in primary total knee replacement. J Bone Joint Surg 2003;85(1):52–6.

28. Järvenpää J, Kettunen J, Kröger H, et al. Obesity may impair the early outcome of total knee arthroplasty a prospective study of 100 patients. Scand J Surg 2010;99(1):45–9.

29. Dorr LD, Boiardo RA. Technical considerations in total knee arthroplasty. Clin Orthop Relat Res 1986;205:5–11.

30. Núñez M, Lozano L, Núñez E, et al. Good quality of life in severely obese total knee replacement patients: a case-control study. Obes Surg 2011;21(8): 1203–8.

31. Chee YH, Teoh KH, Sabnis BM, et al. Total hip replacement in morbidly obese patients with osteoarthritis. J Bone Joint Surg Br 2010;92(8):1066–71.

32. Mechanick JI, Youdim A, Jones DB, et al. Clinical practice guidelines for the perioperative nutritional, metabolic, and nonsurgical support of the bariatric surgery patient—2013 update: Cosponsored by American Association of Clinical Endocrinologists, The Obesity Society, and American Society for Metabolic & Bariatric Surgery. Obesity 2013; 21(S1):S1–27.

33. Chang S-H, Stoll CRT, Song J, et al. The effectiveness and risks of bariatric surgery: an updated systematic review and meta-analysis, 2003-2012. JAMA Surg 2014;149(3):275.

34. Zhang Y, Ju W, Sun X, et al. Laparoscopic sleeve gastrectomy versus laparoscopic Roux-en-Y gastric bypass for morbid obesity and related comorbidities: a meta-analysis of 21 studies. Obes Surg 2015;25(1):19–26.

35. Gill RS, Al-Adra DP, Shi X, et al. The benefits of bariatric surgery in obese patients with hip and knee osteoarthritis: a systematic review. Obes Rev 2011;12(12):1083–9.

36. Groen VA, van de Graaf VA, Scholtes VAB, et al. Effects of bariatric surgery for knee complaints in (morbidly) obese adult patients: a systematic review: bariatric surgery for knee complaints. Obes Rev 2015;16(2):161–70.

37. Bergmann G, Graichen F, Rohlmann A, editors. Implantable telemetry in orthopaedics: workshop: papers. Berlin: Freie Universität; 1990.

38. Abu-Abeid S, Wishnitzer N, Szold A, et al. The influence of surgically-induced weight loss on the knee joint. Obes Surg 2005;15(10):1432–42.

39. Hooper MM, Stellato TA, Hallowell PT, et al. Musculoskeletal findings in obese subjects before and after weight loss following bariatric surgery. Int J Obes 2007;31(1):114–20.

40. Vincent HK, Ben-David K, Conrad BP, et al. Rapid changes in gait, musculoskeletal pain, and quality of life after bariatric surgery. Surg Obes Relat Dis 2012;8(3):346–54.

41. Vartiainen P, Bragge T, Lyytinen T, et al. Kinematic and kinetic changes in obese gait in bariatric surgery-induced weight loss. J Biomech 2012; 45(10):1769–74.

42. Trofa D, Smith EL, Shah V, et al. Total weight loss associated with increased physical activity after bariatric surgery may increase the need for total joint arthroplasty. Surg Obes Relat Dis 2014;10(2): 335–9.

43. Chapman N, Hill K, Taylor S, et al. Patterns of physical activity and sedentary behavior after bariatric surgery: an observational study. Surg Obes Relat Dis 2014;10(3):524–30.

44. Afshar S, Seymour K, Kelly SB, et al. Changes in physical activity after bariatric surgery: using objective and self-reported measures. Surg Obes Relat Dis 2017;13(3):474–83.

45. Fortin PR, Clarke AE, Joseph L, et al. Outcomes of total hip and knee replacement. Arthritis Rheum 1999;42(8):1722–8.

46. Werner BC, Kurkis GM, Gwathmey FW, et al. Bariatric surgery prior to total knee arthroplasty is associated with fewer postoperative complications. J Arthroplasty 2015;30(9):81–5.

47. Kulkarni A, Jameson SS, James P, et al. Does bariatric surgery prior to lower limb joint replacement reduce complications? Surgeon 2011;9(1):18–21.

48. Severson EP, Singh JA, Browne JA, et al. Total knee arthroplasty in morbidly obese patients treated with bariatric surgery. J Arthroplasty 2012;27(9):1696–700.

49. Inacio MCS, Paxton EW, Fisher D, et al. Bariatric surgery prior to total joint arthroplasty may not provide dramatic improvements in post-arthroplasty surgical outcomes. J Arthroplasty 2014;29(7):1359–64.

50. Martin JR, Watts CD, Taunton MJ. Bariatric surgery does not improve outcomes in patients undergoing primary total joint arthroplasty. Bone Joint J 2015;97-B:1501–5.

51. Sjöström L, Peltonen M, Jacobson P, et al. Bariatric surgery and long-term cardiovascular events. J Am Med Assoc 2012;308(1):56–65.

52. Hurwit DJ, Trehan SK, Cross MB. New joints, same old weight: weight changes after total hip and knee arthroplasty. HSS J 2016;12(2):193–5.

53. Dowsey MM, Liew D, Stoney JD, et al. The impact of pre-operative obesity on weight change and outcome in total knee replacement. Bone Joint J 2010;92(4):513–20.

54. Wadden TA, Sarwer DB, Berkowitz RI. Behavioural treatment of the overweight patient. Best Pract Res Clin Endocrinol Metab 1999;13(1):93–107.

55. Ozer K, Abdelnour S, Alva AS. The importance of caloric restriction in the early improvements in insulin sensitivity after Roux-en-Y gastric bypass surgery: comment on Isbell et al. Diabetes Care 2010;33(12):e176.

56. Walls JD, Abraham D, Nelson CL, et al. Hypoalbuminemia more than morbid obesity is an independent predictor of complications after total hip arthroplasty. J Arthroplasty 2015;30(12):2290–5.

57. Nelson CL, Elkassabany NM, Kamath AF, et al. Low albumin levels, more than morbid obesity, are associated with complications after TKA. Clin Orthopaedics Relat Res 2015;473(10):3163–72.

58. Fielden JM, Cumming JM, Horne JG, et al. Waiting for hip arthroplasty. J Arthroplasty 2005;20(8):990–7.

59. Bronson WH, Fewer M, Godlewski K, et al. The ethics of patient risk modification prior to elective joint replacement surgery. J Bone Joint Surg Am 2014;96(13):e113.

60. Klifto K, Klifto C, Slover J. Current concepts of shared decision making in orthopedic surgery. Curr Rev Musculoskelet Med 2017;10(2):253–7.

61. Tarride JE, Haq M, O'Reilly DJ, et al. The excess burden of osteoarthritis in the province of Ontario. Arthritis Rheum 2012;64(14):1153–61.

62. Culler SD, Jevsevar DS, Shea KG, et al. The incremental hospital cost and length-of-stay associated with treating adverse events among Medicare beneficiaries undergoing THA during fiscal year 2013. J Arthroplasty 2016;31(1):42–8.

63. Culler SD, Jevsevar DS, McGuire KJ, et al. Predicting the incremental hospital cost of adverse events among Medicare beneficiaries in the comprehensive joint replacement program during fiscal year 2014. J Arthroplasty 2017;32(6):1732–8.e1.

64. Flego A, Dowsey MM, Choong PFM, et al. Addressing obesity in the management of knee and hip osteoarthritis: weighing in from an economic perspective. BMC Musculoskelet Disord 2016;17(1):233.

65. Dimick JB. Does bariatric surgery reduce health care costs?: weighing the evidence. JAMA Surg 2015;150(8):795.

66. Lewis KH, Zhang F, Arterburn DE, et al. Comparing medical costs and use after laparoscopic adjustable gastric banding and Roux-en-Y gastric bypass. JAMA Surg 2015;150(8):787.

67. McLawhorn AS, Southren D, Wang YC, et al. Cost-effectiveness of bariatric surgery prior to total knee arthroplasty in the morbidly obese: a computer model-based evaluation. J Bone Joint Surg 2016;98(2):e6.

Trauma

Trauma

Obesity in the Polytrauma Patient

Clay A. Spitler, MD*, R. Miles Hulick, MD, Matthew L. Graves, MD,
George V. Russell, MD, Patrick F. Bergin, MD

KEYWORDS

- Obesity • Polytrauma • Resuscitation • Fracture care

KEY POINTS

- Obesity in the United States has reached epidemic status and obesity negatively affects outcomes of patients with trauma.
- Obese patients with trauma have unique physiologic differences that make initial resuscitation more difficult and less effective than resuscitation in normal-weight patients.
- Fracture care in the obese is considerably more difficult because of the size and depth of surgical dissection needed. The obese have higher rates of wound complication, deep infection, failure of fixation, and nonunion.
- Obese patients with polytrauma have higher rates of multiorgan failure and mortality.
- As obesity rates increase, the rates of obesity in patients with trauma increase, and trauma care must continue to develop more effective ways to treat these complicated patients.

INTRODUCTION

Epidemiology

Obesity is an epidemic showing no sign of slowing down and the prevalence has more than doubled worldwide since 1980.[1–3] Obesity is most commonly measured by the body mass index (BMI), and the US Centers for Disease Control and Prevention define obesity as BMI greater than 30 kg/m,[2] with BMI greater than 40 kg/m2 characterized as extreme or morbid obesity. In 2014, more than 600 million people worldwide (13%) were classified as obese and rates of obesity in the United States are among the highest in the world. Between the years 2011 to 2014, the prevalence of obesity reached 36% of the total population of the United States.[1–3] As western populations grow, rates of obesity in patients with trauma will continue to grow with it. This article describes the altered physiology of obese patients with trauma and some of the unique difficulties of caring for these patients.

Burden of Disease

Obesity is a component of the diagnosis of metabolic syndrome, and is a risk factor for cardiovascular disease, stroke, diabetes, and multiple forms of cancer. Increased BMI is also a major risk factor for the development of osteoarthritis.[2] Obesity has created a significant health burden in the United States, with an estimated 300,000 deaths annually caused by obesity, which is 3 times the number of deaths caused by colon and breast cancers combined.[4,5] Accordingly, obesity is considered the leading cause of preventable death, outranking both tobacco and alcohol use.[6] A 25-year-old morbidly obese man has a 22% decreased life expectancy

Disclosure: C.A. Spitler has received research grants from DePuy Synthes, has received honoraria for resident teaching from AO North America, and serves on the OTA EBVQS and AAOS OKU committee. R.M. Hulick has nothing to disclose. M.L. Graves is a design consultant and speaker for Depuy Synthes. G.V. Russell, MD, is a shareholder of Zimmer stock and has a consulting relationship with SMV Orthopedic Implants.
Department of Orthopaedic Surgery, University of Mississippi Medical Center, 2500 North State Street, Jackson, MS 39216, USA
* Corresponding author.
E-mail address: clayspitler@yahoo.com

compared with a man of normal size, correlating to 12 years of life lost.[4]

In addition to the general negative health effects related to obesity, population studies indicate that obese patients are at a 48% increased risk of trauma, including fractures.[7] Obese workers are more likely to sustain workplace injuries and the overall direct cost of care to employers increases with higher BMI of the injured worker.[8] This fining is especially discouraging because this patient group has the lowest overall baseline productivity.[9]

The annual cost of care for obesity and obesity-related conditions in the United States is estimated to be approximately $190 billion, which is about 21% of all US health care expenditure.[9] The average increased cost of medical care for an obese individual is approximately $1500 more per year and more than $39,000 over the course of a lifetime.[9] As obesity prevalence increases, the cost to the US health care economy can be expected to increase as well.

Basic Science

Adipose tissue acts as an energy storage depot but also has unique endocrine, immune, cardiovascular, and metabolic functions. Adipocytes undergo morphologic and metabolic alterations/regulation in the setting of trauma and critical illness, although the understanding of these changes continues to evolve. Adipokines, a class of hormones, are produced by adipocytes and these hormones are directly involved in the regulation of overall adipose tissue mass through the central nervous system and indirectly involved with other hormonal processes like glycemic control through their interaction with insulin and glucagon.[10] Obese and overweight patients have increased baseline levels of inflammation with increased levels of inflammatory markers like C-reactive protein,[11] and adipokines are thought to be one of the primary causes of this chronic inflammation.[10,12] Obese patients also have higher concentrations of macrophages in their adipocytes, which secrete inflammatory cytokines like interleukin-6 and tumor necrosis factor alpha.[13] Chronic exposure to these inflammatory cytokines contributes to the metabolic syndrome, chronic insulin resistance, atherogenic dyslipidemia, hypertriglyceridemia, hyperleptinemia, cardiac disease, and endothelial dysfunction commonly seen in obese patients.

Adipokines also affect regulation of bone cell function and bone structure, and are implicated in the biochemical processes involved in the development of osteoarthritis.[14] Leptin, the most well-described adipokine, is found in significantly higher concentrations in the synovial fluid of osteoarthritic joints[15] and is also thought to cause intra-articular inflammation and collagen breakdown.[16–18] This intra-articular inflammation may contribute to impaired healing and recovery following articular fractures in the obese.

Baseline Physiologic Differences in Obese

There are multiple ways that the physiology of the obese is different from that of normal-weight patients both at baseline and in response to trauma. Respiratory differences in the obese include higher ventilation demands (because of higher systemic oxygen demands), increased work of breathing (because of the force required to move the ribcage and displace intra-abdominal fat), increased airway resistance, and decreased respiratory compliance.[19] In addition, the obese have higher rates of obstructive sleep apnea and reactive airway disease, which can complicate airway management. Cardiovascular differences in the obese include higher resting heart rates and difficulty in increasing left ventricular ejection fraction because of higher peripheral resistance. These changes lead to ventricular hypertrophy and diastolic dysfunction when present over a long period of time.[20] Atherosclerosis commonly occurs with obesity-related comorbidities and contributes to both coronary artery and peripheral vascular disease. Obese patients are at significantly higher risk of thromboembolic events at baseline because of endothelial cell changes, platelet dysfunction, and the release of prothrombotic cytokines from adipose tissue, and this risk is amplified after trauma.[8]

Obesity has well-documented associations with diabetes mellitus and hypertension, which are the most common causes of kidney disease, but obesity has also been found to be an independent risk factor for kidney dysfunction.[21] Obesity also disrupts the integrity of the immune system and leads to alterations in white blood cell development, migration, and diversity. The inflammation associated with obesity seems to blunt the immune response to trauma and pathogens. Obese people have increased absolute numbers of inflammatory leukocytes but show overall impaired ability to mount an immune response.[22]

By application of Wolff's law, the increased forces seen in the weight-bearing extremities of the obese commonly lead to higher bone density. In spite of the reality that absolute bone density is higher in the obese population, this effect disappears when the values are adjusted by BMI.[12,23] The marginal increase in bone density likely does not compensate for the increased loads placed across the skeleton enough to decrease or prevent fractures, primarily because of the momentum generated by the larger mass of obese patients. This point is particularly relevant in seemingly low-energy falls from standing.[12,23]

Preoperative Concerns
Injury patterns
Over the course of their lives, patients with a BMI 25 to 30 have a 15% increased odds of sustaining an injury, and up to 48% increased odds with a BMI greater than 40 compared with patients of normal BMI.[23–26] The severity of both soft tissue injuries and fractures seen in the obese population is higher because of the increased energy associated with larger body size.[25,27,28] In both blunt and penetrating trauma, the soft tissue envelope of obese patients may be protective of visceral injuries, but, because the energy is transmitted to the axial and appendicular osseous structures, these patients are also more likely to sustain injuries to the pelvis,[29] distal femur,[30] ankle,[31] and calcaneus.[23]

In the obese population, low-energy mechanisms often result in high-energy fracture patterns.[12,23,24,28] Knee dislocations secondary to low-energy trauma occur more frequently in obese persons.[12,23,32] A high prevalence of associated popliteal artery injury in this population leads to a higher rate of complications and a higher rate of above-knee amputation compared with patients of normal weight.[12,23,33] Because of the higher level of body mass, fractures of the distal aspect of long bones are at risk for higher levels of comminution.[30] However, the cushioning effect of central obesity may have a protective effect for some fractures, because obese postmenopausal women report falling more often but have fewer hip fractures.[34]

Resuscitation
Prehospital care presents unique challenges in the obese, with greater difficulty in patient transport, noninvasive monitoring, intravenous access, and airway control, which are impeded by the patient's size.[8,35,36] On arrival at the emergency department, obese patients with trauma, on average, have higher base deficits than similarly injured normal-weight patients[37] and during resuscitation they are often under-resuscitated when fluid and blood product administration is not adjusted for their larger size.[38,39] However,

in the morbidly obese who are appropriately resuscitated, acidosis resolves much more slowly than in normal-weight patients even after cardiovascular stability has been achieved.[37,39] Glycemic control, which can also be an important factor in patient outcomes after trauma, is more difficult to manage in the obese because of their higher likelihood of insulin resistance.[40] Ultimately these and other factors lead to higher rates of multiorgan failure and mortality after trauma in obese patients.

Imaging
Imaging protocols for plain radiographs, computed tomography (CT), and MRI must be altered in order to improve the quality of imaging, and poor-quality imaging caused by overlying soft tissues can contribute to delayed or missed diagnosis of fractures in the obese.[41] In addition, the physical limitations of the CT table can preclude safe use in the obese because the weight limit for a standard CT scanner is 202.5 kg (450 lb) and the gantry bore ranges from 80 to 85 cm with a scan field of view ranging from 25 to 82 cm.[42] Specialized scanners for obese patients have an aperture that can accept patients with a waist size of 90 cm.[42] MRI scanners have even more stringent requirements, and obese patients may need to use an open MRI scanner.

Intraoperative Concerns
Positioning/imaging
Standard operating tables typically have 225-kg (500-lb) limits, and the physical dimensions of the bed require additional alterations to safely support the size and weight of some of the largest patients (Fig. 1). Supine positioning in the obese compresses the diaphragm and the inferior vena cava and elevation of the head may be required to safely operate in this

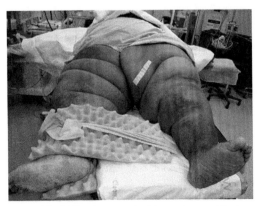

Fig. 1. Morbidly obese patient in supine positioning.

circumstance. Prone positioning can often exacerbate these cardiovascular issues, but lateral positioning is better tolerated and the panniculus is displaced away from the diaphragm and inferior vena cava.[43] Alterations in the anesthetic gases administered can improve postanesthesia recovery by avoiding the more lipophilic gases and calculating anesthetic requirements based on ideal body weight.[24,44,45] Intraoperative fluoroscopy also has limited ability to penetrate large soft tissue envelopes and bony detail can be obscured, making fluoroscopically guided procedures much more difficult.

Fracture care

Upper extremity. Proximal humeral fracture care in those fractures that meet operative indications can be managed with osteosynthesis or arthroplasty, but both options are more difficult because of the larger size of an obese arm. Both the deltopectoral and extended anterolateral approach require a significant amount of retraction/dissection for adequate exposure to surgically treat proximal humeral fractures. In both fixation and arthroplasty there are higher rates of deep infection and postoperative stiffness compared with normal-weight patients.[46]

Nonoperative treatment of diaphyseal humeral fractures is much more difficult in the obese because the size of the chest wall/breast can create unacceptable malalignment and the size of the arm can prevent a functional brace from providing adequate stability. Intramedullary nailing in the obese can be challenging because of limited arm adduction in the obese to allow access to an appropriate starting point. If plating is selected, larger (4.5 mm where possible) and longer plates should be selected in order to provide adequate stability for early mobilization.[24]

In nearly all patients, distal humeral fractures necessitate operative stabilization, but the surgical options in the obese are limited. Total elbow arthroplasty typically requires a lifetime of limited weight bearing and is poorly tolerated in the obese, who commonly require the use of their upper extremities to mobilize. Obesity is associated with a higher rate of deep infection, thromboembolic disease (TED), and hardware loosening/breakage in the treatment of distal humeral fractures.[47,48]

Similar to humeral diaphyseal fractures, nonoperative treatment of distal radius fractures is challenging because of difficulty in maintaining reduction in a splint/cast. Larger surgical exposures are needed and, as a result, higher rates of soft tissue complications arise in the obese population.[49]

Lower extremity. The goals in treatment of pelvic and acetabular fractures are the same as in normal-weight patients but achieving these goals can be significantly more difficult. In most patients, operative indications in obese pelvic and acetabular fractures should not be altered because of patient size because of the dismal outcomes of nonoperative management of displaced and unstable pelvic and acetabular fractures. Preoperative counseling and meticulous surgical technique can set appropriate expectations and maximize patient outcomes in spite of the increased risks in this population. Morel-Lavelle lesions occur more commonly in the obese because of the larger amount of fat present, and they are more difficult to identify on physical examination because of the volume of fat present in the peritrochanteric region where they most frequently occur.[43]

The depth of surgical dissection and prolonged retraction place open surgical approaches to the pelvis and acetabulum at higher risk of wound complications. Percutaneous fixation of pelvic and acetabular fractures has been suggested as one way to minimize the soft tissue complications in the obese, but it should be noted that bony detail can be significantly obscured on intraoperative fluoroscopy.[50] External fixation provides some stability to the anterior pelvic ring but at the cost of high rates of pin site infection and anterior abdominal impingement. Subcutaneous internal fixation of the anterior pelvic ring has become more popular recently and offers the benefit of no external pin sites but requires an additional surgery for removal and has its own unique complications, including heterotopic bone formation at pin sites, lateral femoral cutaneous nerve injury, and femoral nerve palsy.[51] The rate of complications in pelvic and acetabular surgery increase incrementally as BMI increases. The obese have higher intraoperative blood loss, higher rates of deep infection, higher rates of postoperative TED, and higher rates of loss of reduction. Anatomic articular reduction of the acetabulum becomes more difficult to achieve as patient size increases and morbid obesity is associated with worse reductions.[43,52,53] In spite of the increased risks, open reduction and internal fixation remains the authors' preferred method of treatment of displaced acetabular fractures. Meticulous surgical technique, the use of handheld retractors, frequent retractor repositioning, the liberal use of surgical drains, multilayered closure, use of incisional negative pressure wound therapy, strict glycemic control, and supplemental oxygen can help to minimize wound complications.[43]

Most fractures of the femur from the pertrochanteric to the distal metadiaphysis in the obese population are best treated with load-sharing intramedullary nails in order to protect the entire bone from the supraphysiologic loads seen in the obese and allow early weight bearing. Whenever the fracture pattern allows, retrograde nailing is technically easier than antegrade nailing because of the smaller soft tissue envelope at the knee (**Fig. 2**).[54] Some fractures necessitate antegrade nailing, and the starting guidewire and subsequent reamers for both trochanteric and piriformis nails are easily lateralized by the excessive soft tissue in the obese, which can lead to varus malalignment when the intramedullary implant is placed. Lateral positioning and manual medialization of the guidewire and reamers can help prevent this complication (**Figs. 3** and **4**). Obesity is a risk factor for nonunion, failure of fixation, and deep infection in distal femoral fractures treated with lateral locked plating,[55] which is the most common contemporary method of fixation. In order to maximize implant stability, the authors suggest considering the use of an intramedullary implant combined with a plate or dual plating of the distal femur in order to allow the construct to withstand the supraphysiologic loads seen in the obese.

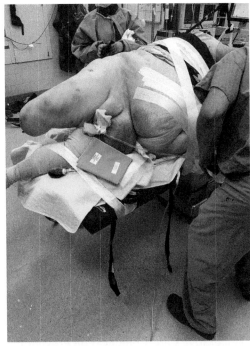

Fig. 3. Morbidly obese patient with a pertrochanteric femur fracture treated with a cephalomedullary nail in the lateral position.

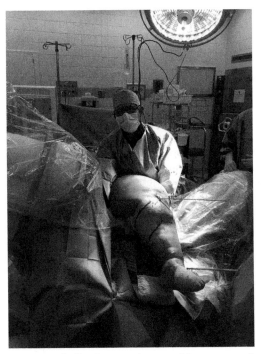

Fig. 2. Morbidly obese patient receiving retrograde nailing.

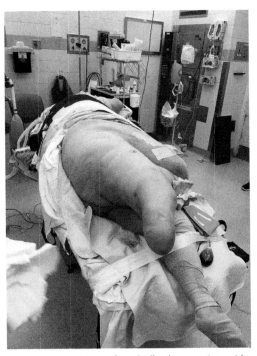

Fig. 4. Posterior view of morbidly obese patient with a pertrochanteric femur fracture treated with a cephalomedullary nail in the lateral position.

Fractures of the tibia in the obese present similar challenges and have similar complication profiles to fractures of the femur. Higher wound complication and infection rates are seen in periarticular and diaphyseal tibial fractures and higher rates of nonunion occur in both plate fixation and intramedullary nailing of tibial fractures in obese patients.[56,57] In the obese, medical complications occur more frequently, hospital stays are longer, and use of inpatient rehabilitation and skilled nursing facilities is higher after lower extremity fractures, in large part because of the difficulty mobilizing after fracture fixation.[56] Loss of reduction is a serious complication in rotational ankle fractures and occurs more frequently in the obese. Failure of fixation in ankle fractures is also closely associated with peripheral neuropathy and diabetes, which are commonly associated with obesity.[58] Fixation in the obese should be maximized and periods of non–weight bearing increased to potentially decrease failure rates.

Postoperative Care/Complication Prevention

The obese have unique postoperative needs and have higher rates of perioperative complications than normal-weight patients. The obese benefit from continuous passive airway pressure and aggressive respiratory therapy to help maintain lung inflation in spite of large amounts of truncal obesity.[39,59] In spite of improving trauma care, the obese continue to have a higher risk of pneumonia and remain in the intensive care unit (ICU) longer than the nonobese.[60–62] Multimodal analgesia and regional anesthetic blocks should be used to maximize pain control while minimizing opioid use (and associated respiratory depression) wherever possible.[24,63]

Obesity has been identified as an independent risk factor for kidney injury.[21] The obese are predisposed to perioperative kidney injury caused by common preexisting kidney disease, preoperative fasting, and increased urine output caused by diabetic and antihypertensive medications. In addition, increased peripheral vascular resistance in the obese may lead to decreased perfusion of the kidneys and other end organs. A delicate balance must be struck between increased fluid resuscitation to perfuse end organs and the ability of the obese patient's diseased heart to compensate for the additional fluid.[21] In spite of improved understanding of the physiology of the obese, they remain at significantly higher risk for multiorgan failure after trauma.[35,38,39,61,64]

The risk of thromboembolic disease is twice as high in obese patients. Pulmonary hypertension, chronic inflammation, and impaired fibrinolysis increase the risk of TED at baseline in the obese, and venous stasis caused by limited mobility in patients with trauma makes this risk significantly higher than in normal-weight patients.[4,65] Early mobilization, mechanical prophylaxis, and use of unfractionated heparin or low-molecular-weight heparin with weight-based dosing should be used to mitigate this increased risk.

Trauma care has improved significantly over the last 2 decades, but obesity remains an independent risk factor for mortality after trauma.[35,61,66] Compared with normal-weight patients of identical injury severity, obese patients have higher rates of all complications, longer ICU stays, and higher rates of mortality.[67] Trauma continues to be the most common cause of death in the United States in patients from 1 to 45 years old, and obesity rates continue to increase at a record pace. Further basic science and clinical research is needed to improve outcomes and decrease mortality in obese patients with trauma. Those patients who do survive face higher rates of wound healing complications, longer hospital stays, and are more likely to require admission to skilled nursing facilities after discharge.[64,68] They progress in rehabilitation more slowly, achieve poorer functional status, and have higher rates of nonunion.[69,70]

SUMMARY

The rates of obesity continue to increase in the United States and the overall impact of obesity on health care spending and patient outcomes after trauma is considerable. The unique physiology of the obese places them at higher risk for complications, including infection, nonunion, multiorgan failure, and death. These physiologic changes and overall patient size can make orthopedic care in obese patients with trauma more difficult, but appropriate initial resuscitation, careful preoperative planning, meticulous surgical technique, diligent postoperative medical management, and specialized rehabilitation give these patients their best opportunity for a good outcome.

REFERENCES

1. Centers for Disease Control and Prevention. Defining adult overweight and obesity. Available at: https://www.cdc.gov/obesity/adult/defining.html. Accessed November 18, 2017.
2. World Health Organization. 10 facts on obesity. Available at: http://www.who.int/features/factfiles/obesity/en/. Accessed November 18, 2017.

3. Ogden CL, Carroll MD, Fryar CD, et al. Prevalence of obesity among adults and youth: United States, 2011-2014. NCHS Data Brief 2015;(219):1–8.

4. Richards WO. Morbid obesity. In: Townsend CM, Beauchamp RD, Evers BM, et al, editors. Sabiston textbook of surgery. 19th edition. Philadelphia: Elsevier Saunders; 2012. p. 358.

5. Mokdad AH, Marks JS, Stroup DF, et al. Actual causes of death in the United States, 2000. JAMA 2004;291(10):1238–45.

6. Sturm R. The effects of obesity, smoking, and drinking on medical problems and costs. Health Aff (Millwood) 2002;21(2):245–53.

7. Acosta-Olivo C, Gonzalez-Saldivar JC, Villarreal-Villarreal G, et al. Correlation between obesity and severity of distal radius fractures. Orthop Traumatol Surg Res 2017;103(2):199–202.

8. Greenberger S, Werman HA. Obesity in trauma care. Trauma Rep 2014. Available at: https://www.ahcmedia.com/articles/31411-obesity-in-trauma-care. Accessed January 29, 2018.

9. Hruby A, Hu F. The epidemiology of obesity: a big picture. Pharmacoecomonics 2015;33(7):673–89.

10. Mittwede PN, Clemmer JS, Bergin PF, et al. Obesity and critical illness: insights from animal models. Shock 2016;45(4):349–58.

11. Visser M, Bouter LM, McQuillan GM, et al. Elevated C-reactive protein levels in overweight and obese adults. JAMA 1999;282(22):2131–5.

12. Parratte S, Pesenti S, Argenson JN. Obesity in orthopedics and trauma surgery. Orthop Traumatol Surg Res 2014;100(1 Suppl):S91–7.

13. Tzanavari T, Giannogonas P, Karalis KP. TNF-alpha and obesity. Curr Dir Autoimmun 2010;11:145–56.

14. Berry PA, Jones SW, Cicuttini FM, et al. Temporal relationship between serum adipokines, biomarkers of bone and cartilage turnover, and cartilage volume loss in a population with clinical knee osteoarthritis. Arthritis Rheum 2011;63(3):700–7.

15. Simopoulou T, Malizos KN, Iliopoulos D, et al. Differential expression of leptin and leptin's receptor isoform (Ob-Rb) mRNA between advanced and minimally affected osteoarthritic cartilage; effect on cartilage metabolism. Osteoarthritis Cartilage 2007;15(8):872–83.

16. Figenschau Y, Knutsen G, Shahazeydi S, et al. Human articular chondrocytes express functional leptin receptors. Biochem Biophys Res Commun 2001;287(1):190–7.

17. Otero M, Gomez Reino JJ, Gualillo O. Synergistic induction of nitric oxide synthase type II: in vitro effect of leptin and interferon-gamma in human chondrocytes and ATDC5 chondrogenic cells. Arthritis Rheum 2003;48(2):404–9.

18. Otero M, Lago R, Lago F, et al. Signalling pathway involved in nitric oxide synthase type II activation in chondrocytes: synergistic effect of leptin with interleukin-1. Arthritis Res Ther 2005;7(3):R581–91.

19. Parameswaran K, Todd DC, Soth M. Altered respiratory physiology in obesity. Can Respir J 2006;13(4):203–10.

20. Vasan RS. Cardiac function and obesity. Heart 2003;89(10):1127–9.

21. Wickman C, Kramer H. Obesity and kidney disease: potential mechanisms. Semin Nephrol 2013;33(1):14–22.

22. Andersen CJ, Murphy KE, Fernandez ML. Impact of obesity and metabolic syndrome on immunity. Adv Nutr 2016;7(1):66–75.

23. Sabharwal S, Root MZ. Impact of obesity on orthopaedics. J Bone Joint Surg Am 2012;94(11):1045–52.

24. Jones CB. Management of upper extremity injuries in obese patients. Orthop Clin North Am 2011;42(1):11–9, v.

25. Streubel PN, Gardner MJ, Ricci WM. Management of femur shaft fractures in obese patients. The Orthop Clin North America 2011;42(1):21–35, v.

26. Finkelstein EA, Chen H, Prabhu M, et al. The relationship between obesity and injuries among U.S. adults. Am J Health Promot 2007;21(5):460–8.

27. Sems SA, Johnson M, Cole PA, et al, Minnesota Orthopaedic Trauma Group. Elevated body mass index increases early complications of surgical treatment of pelvic ring injuries. J Orthop Trauma 2010;24(5):309–14.

28. Graves ML, Porter SE, Fagan BC, et al. Is obesity protective against wound healing complications in pilon surgery? Soft tissue envelope and pilon fractures in the obese. Orthopedics 2010;33(8).

29. Bansal V, Conroy C, Lee J, et al. Is bigger better? The effect of obesity on pelvic fractures after side impact motor vehicle crashes. J Trauma 2009;67(4):709–14.

30. Maheshwari R, Mack CD, Kaufman RP, et al. Severity of injury and outcomes among obese trauma patients with fractures of the femur and tibia: a crash injury research and engineering network study. J Orthop Trauma 2009;23(9):634–9.

31. Strauss EJ, Frank JB, Walsh M, et al. Does obesity influence the outcome after the operative treatment of ankle fractures? J Bone Joint Surg Br 2007;89(6):794–8.

32. Peltola EK, Lindahl J, Hietaranta H, et al. Knee dislocation in overweight patients. AJR Am J Roentgenol 2009;192(1):101–6.

33. Hagino RT, DeCaprio JD, Valentine RJ, et al. Spontaneous popliteal vascular injury in the morbidly obese. J Vasc Surg 1998;28(3):458–62 [discussion: 462–3].

34. Beck TJ, Petit MA, Wu G, et al. Does obesity really make the femur stronger? BMD, geometry, and fracture incidence in the women's health initiative-

observational study. J Bone Miner Res 2009;24(8): 1369–79.

35. Hoffmann M, Lefering R, Gruber-Rathmann M, et al, Trauma Registry of the German Society for Trauma C. The impact of BMI on polytrauma outcome. Injury 2012;43(2):184–8.

36. Sakles JC, Patanwala AE, Mosier JM, et al. Comparison of video laryngoscopy to direct laryngoscopy for intubation of patients with difficult airway characteristics in the emergency department. Intern Emerg Med 2014;9(1):93–8.

37. Rae L, Pham TN, Carrougher G, et al. Differences in resuscitation in morbidly obese burn patients may contribute to high mortality. J Burn Care Res 2013;34(5):507–14.

38. Nelson J, Billeter AT, Seifert B, et al. Obese trauma patients are at increased risk of early hypovolemic shock: a retrospective cohort analysis of 1,084 severely injured patients. Crit Care 2012;16(3):R77.

39. Winfield RD, Delano MJ, Lottenberg L, et al. Traditional resuscitative practices fail to resolve metabolic acidosis in morbidly obese patients after severe blunt trauma. J Trauma 2010;68(2):317–30.

40. Sperry JL, Frankel HL, Nathens AB, et al. Characterization of persistent hyperglycemia: what does it mean postinjury? J Trauma 2009;66(4):1076–82.

41. Laasonen EM, Kivioja A. Delayed diagnosis of extremity injuries in patients with multiple injuries. J Trauma 1991;31(2):257–60.

42. Modica MJ, Kanal KM, Gunn ML. The obese emergency patient: imaging challenges and solutions. Radiographics 2011;31(3):811–23.

43. Gettys FK, Russell GV, Karunakar MA. Open treatment of pelvic and acetabular fractures. The Orthop Clin North America 2011;42(1):69–83, vi.

44. Domi R, Laho H. Anesthetic challenges in the obese patient. J Anesth 2012;26(5):758–65.

45. Peters A, Kerner W. Perioperative management of the diabetic patient. Exp Clin Endocrinol Diabetes 1995;103(4):213–8.

46. Werner BC, Griffin JW, Yang S, et al. Obesity is associated with increased postoperative complications after operative management of proximal humerus fractures. J Shoulder Elbow Surg 2015; 24(4):593–600.

47. Werner BC, Rawles RB, Jobe JT, et al. Obesity is associated with increased postoperative complications after operative management of distal humerus fractures. J Shoulder Elbow Surg 2015;24(10): 1602–6.

48. Claessen FM, Braun Y, Peters RM, et al. Plate and screw fixation of bicolumnar distal humerus fractures: factors associated with loosening or breakage of implants or nonunion. J Hand Surg Am 2015;40(10):2045–51.e2.

49. Fernandez DL. Closed manipulation and casting of distal radius fractures. Hand Clin 2005;21(3):307–16.

50. Bates P, Gary J, Singh G, et al. Percutaneous treatment of pelvic and acetabular fractures in obese patients. The Orthop Clin North America 2011; 42(1):55–67, vi.

51. Chaus G, Weaver M. Anterior subcutaneous internal fixation of the pelvis: placement of the INFIX. Oper Tech Orthopedics 2015;24(4):262–9.

52. Karunakar MA, Shah SN, Jerabek S. Body mass index as a predictor of complications after operative treatment of acetabular fractures. J Bone Joint Surg Am 2005;87(7):1498–502.

53. Porter SE, Russell GV, Dews RC, et al. Complications of acetabular fracture surgery in morbidly obese patients. J Orthop Trauma 2008;22(9): 589–94.

54. Tucker MC, Schwappach JR, Leighton RK, et al. Results of femoral intramedullary nailing in patients who are obese versus those who are not obese: a prospective multicenter comparison study. J Orthop Trauma 2007;21(8):523–9.

55. Ricci WM, Streubel PN, Morshed S, et al. Risk factors for failure of locked plate fixation of distal femur fractures: an analysis of 335 cases. J Orthop Trauma 2014;28(2):83–9.

56. Graves ML. Periarticular tibial fracture treatment in the obese population. The Orthop Clin North America 2011;42(1):37–44, v–vi.

57. Parkkinen M, Madanat R, Lindahl J, et al. Risk factors for deep infection following plate fixation of proximal tibial fractures. J Bone Joint Surg Am 2016;98(15):1292–7.

58. Mendelsohn ES, Hoshino CM, Harris TG, et al. The effect of obesity on early failure after operative syndesmosis injuries. J Orthop Trauma 2013;27(4): 201–6.

59. Andruszkow H, Veh J, Mommsen P, et al. Impact of the body mass on complications and outcome in multiple trauma patients: what does the weight weigh? Mediators Inflamm 2013;2013:345702.

60. Mica L, Keller C, Vomela J, et al. Obesity and overweight as a risk factor for pneumonia in polytrauma patients: a retrospective cohort study. J Trauma Acute Care Surg 2013;75(4):693–8.

61. Bochicchio GV, Joshi M, Bochicchio K, et al. Impact of obesity in the critically ill trauma patient: a prospective study. J Am Coll Surg 2006;203(4):533–8.

62. Serrano PE, Khuder SA, Fath JJ. Obesity as a risk factor for nosocomial infections trauma patients. J Am Coll Surg 2010;211(1):61–7.

63. Guss D, Bhattacharyya T. Perioperative management of the obese orthopaedic patient. J Am Acad Orthop Surg 2006;14(7):425–32.

64. Baldwin KD, Matuszewski PE, Namdari S, et al. Does morbid obesity negatively affect the hospital course of patients undergoing treatment of closed, lower extremity diaphyseal long-bone fractures? Orthopedics 2011;34(1):18.

65. Kornblith LZ, Howard B, Kunitake R, et al. Obesity and clotting: body mass index independently contributes to hypercoagulability after injury. J Trauma Acute Care Surg 2015;78(1):30–6.

66. Wutzler S, Maegele M, Marzi I, et al. Association of preexisting medical conditions with in-hospital mortality in multiple-trauma patients. J Am Coll Surgeons 2009;209(1):75–81.

67. Liu T, Chen JJ, Bai XJ, et al. The effect of obesity on outcomes in trauma patients: a meta-analysis. Injury 2013;44(9):1145–52.

68. Childs BR, Nahm NJ, Dolenc AJ, et al. Obesity is associated with more complications and longer hospital stays after orthopedic trauma. J Orthop Trauma 2015;29(11):504–9.

69. Zura R, Xiong Z, Einhorn T, et al. Epidemiology of fracture nonunion in 18 human bones. JAMA Surg 2016;151(11):e162775.

70. Vincent HK, Seay AN, Vincent KR, et al. Effects of obesity on rehabilitation outcomes after orthopedic trauma. Am J Phys Med Rehabil 2012;91(12):1051–9.

Management of Pelvic and Acetabular Fractures in the Obese Patient

Kevin F. Purcell, MD[a], Patrick F. Bergin, MD[b,*],
Clay A. Spitler, MD[a], Matthew L. Graves, MD[a],
George V. Russell, MD[a]

KEYWORDS

- Pelvic ring • Acetabular fracture • Obese trauma • Fracture management

---

KEY POINTS

- Treatment of acetabular and pelvic ring injuries in the obese population is difficult.
- Preventing complications is crucial in these high-risk, obese trauma patients.
- Patient positioning needs to be meticulous to ensure stability on the bed while allowing access to the operative site, preventing pressure necrosis, and minimizing ventilation pressure.

INTRODUCTION

Pelvic ring and acetabular fractures, in general, are a challenging task for the orthopedic surgeon. Although technically demanding to treat, these injuries become more difficult to manage in the obese population for a myriad of reasons. Preoperative planning is required before bringing the patient to the operating room for fixation of these osseous injuries. It is imperative that the orthopedic surgeon considers the impaired nutritional state, potential anesthetic complications, difficult positioning, limited surgical exposure, challenging rehabilitation, and a myriad of common complications in the obese patient.

It is postulated that by 2030 approximately 80% of the American population will be either overweight or obese.[1] Thus, it is important that

the orthopedic surgeon develop a foundation in managing osseous and other injuries in the obese population. There is significant difficulty in the surgical fixation of acetabular and pelvic ring injuries as well as the perioperative management of obese patients. In this review, we discuss perioperative medical management, intraoperative positioning and techniques, and specific risks of surgery while mitigating potential complications.

EVALUATION AND PREPARATION

It is important that patients who sustain acetabular fractures receive the Advanced Trauma Life Support (ATLS) evaluation. Acetabulum and pelvic ring injuries are high energy in nature, and it would behoove the trauma team to investigate if

---

Disclosure Statement: P.F. Bergin has been a consultant for Synthes and Acumed. He is an Arbeitsgemeinschaft für Osteosynthesefragen (AO) faculty member and has received honoraria for course participation. K.F. Purcell has nothing to disclose. G.V. Russell: American Academy of Orthopaedic Surgeons: Board or committee member; Arbeitsgemeinschaft für Osteosynthesefragen North America - Honoraria for courses: Paid presenter or speaker; Orthopaedic Trauma Association: Board or committee member; SMV: Stock or stock Options. Zimmer: Stock or stock Options. M.L. Graves: Depuy Synthes-design consultant and speaker; Globus Medical-design consultant; SMV- design consultant; AONA and Orthopedic Trauma Association-speaker.
[a] Department of Orthopaedic Surgery and Rehabilitation, University of Mississippi Medical Center (USA), 2500 North State Street, Jackson, MS 39216, USA; [b] Department of Orthopaedic Surgery and Rehabilitation, University of Mississippi Medical Center (USA), 2500 North State Street, Jackson, MS 39216, USA
* Corresponding author.
E-mail address: pbergin@umc.edu

Orthop Clin N Am 49 (2018) 317–324
https://doi.org/10.1016/j.ocl.2018.02.005

there are any other underlying injuries. A dermatologic examination to assess for Morel-Lavallée lesions is especially warranted in the obese population. Given the amount of skin hidden under the panniculus, a thorough examination must be made for open injuries that are commonly missed in the obese patient.[2]

The obese trauma patient often has specific medical problems that must be addressed. Nutritionally, many obese patients are malnourished and suffer from either protein or vitamin deficiencies.[3,4] These nutritional deficiencies in the obese patient may be causally related to the increased morbidity and mortality in this population.[3] It is therefore important that nutritional repletion be considered in obese patients during the preoperative and convalescent phase. In addition, it has been well documented that obese patients have a blunted inflammatory response in an acute trauma setting that could be possibly linked to their increased rate of complications.[5] Specifically, obesity has been linked as an independent risk factor for multiorgan failure even after controlling for confounding factors.[6-8] Obesity has also been linked to an increased rate of death after trauma, and obesity is directly correlated with an increased injury severity score.[9] It should, however, be mentioned that underweight patients also have increased mortality in the polytrauma setting.[10]

It is always important to communicate with the anesthesiology team before bringing any patient to the operating room, but special consideration should be given to the obese patient. Obese patients are more likely to have decreased ability to extend their neck, increased tissue around their oropharynx, and decreased tolerance for tissue hypoxia.[11] There is considerable difficulty with intubating obese patients, especially those with a body mass index (BMI) greater than 40 kg/m^2.[11] Thus, it would be fitting that the anesthesiology team be prepared for difficult intubation and also extubation by having multiple resources at bedside, such as the gum elastic bougie, laryngeal mask airway, or a laryngoscope.

It is important that morbidly obese patients be screened for obstructive sleep apnea (OSA). OSA has been linked to respiratory depression and acute respiratory compromise of obese patients in the perioperative setting.[12] Obese patients are at increased risk for pulmonary complications in the postoperative setting for several reasons.[13] Obese individuals tend to desaturate in the first day postoperatively; however, providing the patient with noninvasive positive pressure ventilation may avoid the postoperative pulmonary complications experienced.[13]

Preventing postoperative hypoxemia should be a vital part of the perioperative management of obese patients.

INITIAL ORTHOPEDIC MANAGEMENT

Urgent stabilization of orthopedic injuries is essential to prevent ongoing soft tissue and bony damage until definitive surgery can be performed. As in lean patients, a concomitant hip dislocation with an acetabular fracture requires urgent closed reduction in the emergency department. Skeletal traction is generally necessary to maintain reduction, decrease pain, and reduce muscle spasms associated with acetabular injuries. However, standard Kirschner wires (K-wires)/Steinman pins may not be long enough to bridge the bone and larger soft tissue envelope. Thus, it is important to measure the wire/pin from the skeletal traction tray to assess if it will traverse the femur/tibia and associated soft tissue envelope. We have used starting wires from intramedullary nail sets as "traction pins" in obese patients when the K-wires were not long enough.

The proper imaging of acetabular and pelvic injuries includes 5 radiographic views (anteroposterior, Judets, Iliac/obturator oblique, inlet, and outlet) and a computed tomography (CT) scan of the pelvis. However, both plain films and advanced imaging of osseous injuries in obese patients are harder to visualize. X-ray photons must pass through a larger soft tissue envelope that increases the amount of time to capture an image.[14] The increase in time can allow motion artifact to obscure the image, and increases the radiation exposure experienced.[14] Standard x-ray machines generally take radiographs by using a preset current (mA) and potential (kVp) depending on the body part. These preset values may not penetrate an obese individual's soft tissue envelope.[14] The inability of x-rays to adequately penetrate tissue increases background scatter.[14] However, if you encounter a situation in which your radiographs are inadequate, you can ask the radiology technologist to increase the mA, kVp, and the image-processing speed. Manipulating these 3 variables can help improve the quality of your radiograph. Also, one can use the Bucky-Potter grid to reduce potential x-ray scatter and increase the resolution of the radiograph.[14]

CT scans are a vital imaging modality used not only in preoperative planning of acetabular fractures and pelvic ring disruptions, but also at times in the postoperative setting to discern if implants violated the articular surface and/or neural foramina during definitive fixation. This is especially true when intraoperative fluoroscopy is limited by bony habitus. CT scan analysis also can be obscured by obesity. The reasoning for this is similar to that of radiographs. Increased tissue attenuates the ability for radiation to penetrate both bone and soft tissue envelope.[14] This can result in increased noise, thus decreasing resolution. Similarly, you can inquire if the radiation technologist can increase the mA/kVp to increase image resolution. Most centers have radiologist technologists who are skilled in increasing the resolution in obese patients, but at times, it helps to give real-time feedback on the quality of studies in challenging patients. Last, there have been instances in which certain obese patients cannot fit in the standard CT scans in the hospital. We have sent patients to the local zoo to use their specialized CT scan and/or MRI equipment to obtain the necessary imaging.

Patient Positioning

A vital part of operating on any patient is considering the operating room (OR) table, patient positioning, and patient safety for the procedure. Obese patients pose a challenge for both selecting OR tables and securing patients once they are on the table. Many OR tables have weight limits, usually approximately 250 kg, that are often exceeded by obese patients. We have used urology cystoscopy tables when operating on morbidly obese patients due to the increased weight limit on these tables that can often be loaded with up to 1000 pounds. When using atypical tables because of the patient's size, we are careful before draping to ensure that we can use fluoroscopy with these tables.

Less often, we combine 2 OR tables to allow the patient's weight to be evenly distributed across a greater surface area. However, this is suboptimal because it can be difficult to use fluoroscopy. Last, there are situations in which we place a stool beneath the operating table to support the additional weight of an obese patient. It is important to be innovative, but practice safe methods while managing obese patients' care in the OR.

Lateral Position

At our center, lateral positioning is generally used for fixation of transverse/posterior wall acetabular fractures with minimal or no anterior column displacement and most posterior wall fractures. This position is often the safest position for the obese patient from a respiratory standpoint, but can be one of the more difficult ways to stabilize the patient on the OR table. For the very large patient in whom ventilation is difficult or even impossible in the prone position, the lateral position offers an opportunity to manage transverse-type fractures that would traditionally be treated with prone approaches. It has been shown that fracture reductions for transverse injuries are often compromised in the lateral relative to the prone position even for lean patients.[15] Unfortunately, the difficulties in managing significant anterior column displacement are often magnified by the weight of the limb, making fracture reduction even more difficult in the obese population.

The abdominal circumference of obese patients generally makes lateral positioning quite challenging. Many OR straps are not long enough to safely secure an obese patient to the OR table. In addition, standard OR beanbags do not safely stabilize the patient on the table. Using an oversized beanbag is the easiest way to stabilize patients in the lateral position, although even they may not extend enough over the panniculus to make a patient stable. We have also combined 2 standard beanbags to stabilize a patient on the OR table or used several straps across the trunk of an obese patient and contralateral leg. It is important to place eggshell foam under the strap to prevent pressure ulcer formation. The lateral position places increased pressure on the bony prominences on the contralateral leg, and it is imperative these areas are padded with additional eggshell foam or padding material.

Supine Position

This position is used for anterior approaches to the acetabulum and pelvic ring. With many of these exposures, a midline bump is helpful both for positioning the pelvis off the bed as well as for allowing the panniculus to retract laterally away from the surgical site. Even when making these bumps wider than usual, the patient can be somewhat unstable. We generally use 2 to 3 chest straps on obese patients to help stabilize them on the bed. We use more straps both for added security as well as to avoid overtightening each individual strap, thus worsening their chest wall compliance. It is unfortunately very easy for these straps to limit diaphragmatic excursion and cause restrictive respiratory compromise. In addition, for supplemental safety, we place ace wraps 3 or 4 times around the nonoperative leg to prevent it from falling off the OR table. If the thighs are too large to allow the legs to stay on stably, an arm board can be added to the distal portion of the bed to help support the leg.

Moreover, it is essential to ensure the panniculus of an obese patient does not enter the sterile field. If the supine position is chosen. There are different maneuvers to ensure the panniculus stays out of the operative field, such as manual retraction of the panniculus during the procedure by an assistant, or taping the panniculus to the contralateral side of the body. There have been instances in which the panniculus has been sutured to the chest wall to make sure that it does not enter the operative field (Figs. 1 and 2). In the very large patient, the panniculus can be brought to the side to prevent overt compression of the chest wall in the supine position. In all instances, reverse Trendelenburg position often helps reduce the ventilation pressure in obese patients. Last, the patient should be monitored for a brief course after prepping the patient on the OR table before making an incision to evaluate the patient for any trouble ventilating due to increased intra-abdominal pressure.

Prone Position

The prone position is notorious for altering the chest physiology in obese patients. There are different measures to decrease the increased intrathoracic and intra-abdominal pressure. We use chest rolls that extend vertically from the anterior superior iliac spine (ASIS) to the thorax. If the patient is not able to ventilate properly with the aforementioned technique, we place chest rolls horizontally across the ASIS and another across the thorax. The chest rolls and foam cushioning should limit the abdomen from pressing against the OR table. Conversely, if both of these techniques fail, then we will fold the panniculus to the nonoperative side to assist with decreasing the intra-abdominal pressure. Last, care must be taken to prevent pressure ulcers and neuropathies in the prone position. A

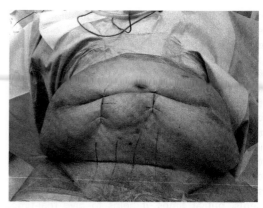

Fig. 2. Panniculus sutured to the chest wall to maintain sterile operative field.

surplus of foam padding should be placed under the knees and feet to decrease pressure on the bony prominences, and foam padding should be placed under the elbows to prevent ulnar neuropathy (**Fig. 3**).

SURGICAL TECHNIQUES
Percutaneous Techniques

Percutaneous fixation of pelvic ring injuries has gained widespread popularity over the recent years. The advantages of percutaneous fixation include decreased blood loss, and infection rate of posterior pelvic ring injuries.[16] However, as in any other surgical procedure, there are risks associated with percutaneous pinning. Routt and colleagues[16] discussed the technical difficulty of obtaining sufficient intraoperative fluoroscopic imaging in the obese patient. This is due to the inability to visualize the sacrum adequately from a lateral image. In addition, sacral anatomy is widely variable from patient to patient. Routt and colleagues[16] elaborated on making larger surgical incisions to place

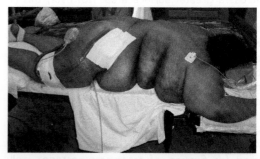

Fig. 3. Obese patient shown in prone position. Chest rolls placed vertically to allow adequate ventilation. Panniculus is folded to the side. At the end of the procedure, an incisional wound VAC is used to help prevent wound complications.

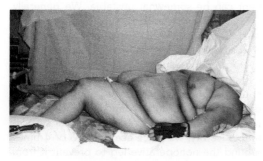

Fig. 1. Morbidly obese patient with panniculus covering operative site.

iliosacral screws. At times, however, longer instruments (eg, guidewires, screwdrivers) can help mitigate this problem.

There are instances in which iliosacral screws may not provide the stability anticipated preoperatively. Transiliac-transsacral screws are a viable option for increased stability in morbidly obese patients.[17] These screws can increase the stability of the construct if the surgeon feels the patient's anatomy allows for placement of these screws. Bates and colleagues[18] elucidated on the difficulty of percutaneous fixation, but strongly promoted this technique as a viable option to mitigate the increased infection and wound complication rate commonly seen in obese patients with open approaches. Lefaivre and colleagues[19] have reported using a pelvic reduction frame to obtain reductions in displaced pelvic ring injuries, and then placing iliosacral screws. For those who are technically proficient with these techniques, this is an option for gaining a reduction of moderately to severely displaced pelvic ring injuries and avoiding the complications of open approaches.

External Fixation

External fixation is an option for managing pelvic ring injuries; however, this option may be quite problematic in the obese population for several reasons. The relatively large soft tissue envelope between the skin and bone allows for motion and breakdown around the pins. Compressive dressings can help prevent some of this motion and extend the life of the half pin but there is a higher pin tract infection rate in obese patients. Biomechanically, the bar is farther away from the bone and therefore the construct is less rigid than in lean peers and care must be taken to create a stable construct despite these limitations. Hupel and colleagues[20] discussed the inability of anterior uniplanar external fixation to maintain stability in open book pelvic ring injuries in the obese population. Conversely, they concluded that plating of the pubic symphysis allowed for earlier mobility and maintained reduction in the postoperative period.[20]

Unfortunately, there is a high incidence of infection with definitive use of external fixation in the obese population.[21] Mason and colleagues[21] conducted a study that showed most of the obese population that was managed definitively with external fixation developed an infection. Thus, it may be an appealing option to use temporarily, but definitive use of external fixation should be cautioned against in obese patients.

The INFIX or internal fixator is another surgical technique that has become an attractive option in managing pelvic ring injuries. The INFIX involves placing a pedicle screw into the supra-acetabular bone in each hemipelvis followed by placement of a subcutaneous bar connecting the screws. The INFIX was created to mitigate the shortcomings of external fixation in obese patients, such as pin tract infections, increased bone to bar distance, and pressure from the panniculus against the external fixation bar.[22] Thus, the INFIX is biomechanically more stable than external fixation in obese patients.

The technique for the INFIX is not overtly challenging, and affords great stability in obese patients although there is a learning curve. Making an incision over the ASIS bilaterally with dissection down to the Sartorius fascia is the initial step in INFIX placement. Subsequently, the rectus femoris is taken down at its origin on the anterior inferior iliac spine. It is important during the aforementioned step to not injure the lateral femoral cutaneous nerve (LFCN) or violate the hip joint capsule. Pedicle screws are then placed in the supra-acetabular region. Last, the connecting bar is placed subcutaneously connecting both pedicle screws. Vaidya and colleagues[22] performed a radiographic review of their early experience with the INFIX and found that most patients healed without loss of reduction. There are complications associated with using the INFIX, including anterior thigh paresthesias secondary to LFCN palsy, heterotopic ossification, and malposition of pedicle screws requiring reoperation.[22,23]

RESULTS/COMPLICATIONS

The literature discussing the functionality of obese patients after fixation of acetabular and pelvic ring injuries is focused mainly on the heightened risk of complications. This is understandable given the extreme complication profile seen with these patients. Although mitigation of complications is important, we need to expand our foundation on how obese patients perform postoperatively.

Porter and colleagues[24] conducted a study at our center that discusses the issues with pelvic ring injury management in the obese population. They found a doubling of complications with a similar doubling of the reoperation rate. Subsequently, Sems and colleagues[25] showed there is a direct relationship between BMI and rate of reoperation and complications after surgical fixation of pelvic ring injuries. Although wound complication is the leading cause of return to the OR in both series, loss of reduction is a complication that is also commonly witnessed in obese patients (**Figs. 4** and **5**). Overall, it has been shown that there is increased time in the OR and higher incidence of infection, deep vein thrombosis (DVT), iatrogenic nerve palsies, and increased reoperation rate after initial surgery for either irrigation and debridement or loss of reduction.[24,25]

Acetabular fracture surgery has similar problems. We have shown at our center that it is often more difficult to attain acetabular reductions in morbidly obese patients.[26] Mears and colleagues[27] presented a similar experience with acetabular fracture reduction. Specifically, they have shown that the most patients with poor reductions had identifiable factors preoperatively that included obesity and femoral neck/head fracture. From a complication standpoint, our center has concluded that obese patients have longer operation times, increased complications, and increased blood loss in comparison with their leaner counterparts.[28] Karunakar and colleagues[29] conducted another study that confirmed our findings. They showed that obese patients had longer operation times, increased prevalence of wound infections, increased DVT rates, and increased instances of extensive blood loss. Specifically, obese

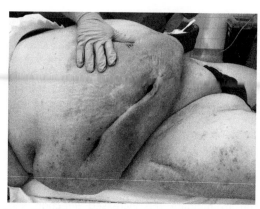

Fig. 5. Wound dehiscence of anterior approach. Please note effort to place incision above panniculus.

patients are 2.6 times more likely to develop a DVT and are 2.1 times more likely to have increased blood loss than their leaner counterparts. In assessing risk factors for deep infection, after open pelvic ring and acetabular fractures, Sagi and colleagues[30] found angio embolization, obesity, and leukocytosis to be independent risk factors. Similarly, there is an increase in complications, such as pneumonia and DVT, even if acetabular/pelvic ring injuries are managed nonoperatively in the obese population.[31] This should serve as an impetus to be meticulous when managing these injuries in obese patients. Every effort must be made to prevent venous thromboembolic disease while also considering blood loss and wound complications.

There is a considerable amount of difficulty with managing these injuries and mitigating complications in the obese population and thus it would seem sensible that there be an increase in reimbursement. We have shown that despite the increased time and effort required to manage obese patients with acetabular fractures that there is no increase in the average reimbursement for operating on morbidly obese patients with these injuries.[32] We have to ask ourselves if this will lead to obese patients with acetabular and pelvic ring injuries being marginalized in the near future. We must serve as advocates to ensure that obese patients receive the same high-quality health care as their leaner counterparts.

Fortunately, we believe there are a few techniques to decrease infection rates in the obese population undergoing surgical fixation. We adhere to sharp dissection through the epidermis, dermis, and adipose layers. Electrocautery should be used for bleeding control, and not for dissecting through the different subcutaneous layers. When using an anterior

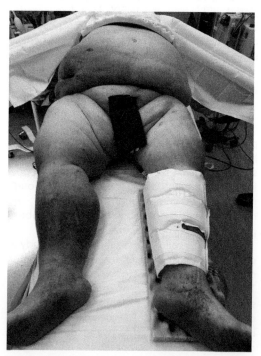

Fig 4 Anterior approach to acetabular fracture with wound dehiscence.

approach to the pelvis, care must be taken to avoid incision around the fold at the inferior aspect of the panniculus. Generally, this area is colonized with microorganisms and has preexisting skin breakdown and it would be appropriate for the surgeon to avoid this area for any incisions. Although making the approach a little more difficult, we try to place the incision a few inches anterior to the nadir of the panniculus fold to avoid this area.

After we place all implants, we resect all necrotic tissue and thoroughly irrigate with saline using a pulsed lavage or cystoscopy tubing. In addition, we place as many Jackson-Pratt drains as necessary in the superficial and deep tissue to ensure a hematoma does not form beneath the surgical incision or implants. We close several layers in the adipose tissue to prevent tissue shearing that can possibly lead to increased bleeding and fat necrosis. We constantly aim to decrease any possible nidus for infection.

Reddix and colleagues[33] strongly advocate for the use of incision vacuum-assisted closure (VAC) devices in morbidly obese patients undergoing acetabular fixation. Their cohort documented no complications, such as infection or surgical incision dehiscence, with VAC devices. Hence, incisional VAC devices serve as another mechanism to assist with decreasing postoperative wound complications. Because of the increased risk of superficial and deep infection in obese patients, there should be a low threshold for returning to the OR for an irrigation and debridement. Our personal philosophy is to return to the OR for debridement if there is persistent drainage 1 week out from surgery. Although this has not been studied to prevent deep infections, we do believe that aggressive complication management is warranted.

Last, we educate all patients, especially our obese patients, on the significance of mobilizing with physical therapy and the use of incentive spirometry postoperatively. There is increased risk of DVT and pneumonia in obese patients undergoing pelvic ring/acetabular fixation and every action must be taken to decrease these complications from occurring.[31]

SUMMARY

Treatment of acetabular and pelvic ring injuries in the obese population is technically difficult and fraught with an increase in the complication rate. There are numerous factors to consider in preventing complications in these high-risk patients. We must ensure that patients are receiving high-quality health care and being judiciously monitored to minimize complications and aggressively manage those that occur.

REFERENCES

1. Wang Y, Beydoun MA, Liang L, et al. Will all Americans become overweight or obese? Estimating the progression and cost of the US obesity epidemic. Obesity (Silver Spring) 2008;16(10):2323–30.
2. Gettys FK, Russell GV, Karunakar MA. Open treatment of pelvic and acetabular fractures. Orthop Clin North Am 2011;42(1):69–83, vi.
3. Davidson LJ, Bennett SE, Hamera EK, et al. What constitutes advanced assessment? J Nurs Educ 2004;43(9):421–5.
4. Elamin EM. Nutritional care of the obese intensive care unit patient. Curr Opin Crit Care 2005;11(4):300–3.
5. Winfield RD, Delano MJ, Cuenca AG, et al. Obese patients show a depressed cytokine profile following severe blunt injury. Shock 2012;37(3):253–6.
6. Ciesla DJ, Moore EE, Johnson JL, et al. Obesity increases risk of organ failure after severe trauma. J Am Coll Surg 2006;203(4):539–45.
7. Edmonds RD, Cuschieri J, Minei JP, et al. Body adipose content is independently associated with a higher risk of organ failure and nosocomial infection in the nonobese patient postinjury. J Trauma 2011;70(2):292–8.
8. Brown CV, Neville AL, Rhee P, et al. The impact of obesity on the outcomes of 1,153 critically injured blunt trauma patients. J Trauma 2005;59(5):1048–51 [discussion: 1051].
9. Byrnes MC, McDaniel MD, Moore MB, et al. The effect of obesity on outcomes among injured patients. J Trauma 2005;58(2):232–7.
10. Hoffmann M, Lefering R, Gruber-Rathmann M, et al, Trauma Registry of the German Society for Trauma Surgery. The impact of BMI on polytrauma outcome. Injury 2012;43(2):184–8.
11. Holmberg TJ, Bowman SM, Warner KJ, et al. The association between obesity and difficult prehospital tracheal intubation. Anesth Analg 2011;112(5):1132–8.
12. Benumof JL. Obstructive sleep apnea in the adult obese patient: implications for airway management. Anesthesiol Clin North America 2002;20(4):789–811.
13. Neligan PJ, Malhotra G, Fraser M, et al. Noninvasive ventilation immediately after extubation improves lung function in morbidly obese patients with obstructive sleep apnea undergoing laparoscopic bariatric surgery. Anesth Analg 2010;110(5):1360–5.

14. Uppot RN, Sahani DV, Hahn PF, et al. Impact of obesity on medical imaging and image-guided intervention. AJR Am J Roentgenol 2007;188(2): 433–40.

15. Collinge C, Archdeacon M, Sagi HC. Quality of radiographic reduction and perioperative complications for transverse acetabular fractures treated by the Kocher-Langenbeck approach: prone versus lateral position. J Orthop Trauma 2011;25(9): 538–42.

16. Routt ML Jr, Simonian PT, Mills WJ. Iliosacral screw fixation: early complications of the percutaneous technique. J Orthop Trauma 1997;11(8):584–9.

17. Gardner MJ, Routt ML Jr. Transiliac-transsacral screws for posterior pelvic stabilization. J Orthop Trauma 2011;25(6):378–84.

18. Bates P, Gary J, Singh G, et al. Percutaneous treatment of pelvic and acetabular fractures in obese patients. Orthop Clin North America 2011;42(1): 55–67, vi.

19. Lefaivre KA, Starr AJ, Barker BP, et al. Early experience with reduction of displaced disruption of the pelvic ring using a pelvic reduction frame. J Bone Joint Surg Br 2009;91(9):1201–7.

20. Hupel TM, McKee MD, Waddell JP, et al. Primary external fixation of rotationally unstable pelvic fractures in obese patients. J Trauma 1998;45(1): 111–5.

21. Mason WT, Khan SN, James CL, et al. Complications of temporary and definitive external fixation of pelvic ring injuries. Injury 2005;36(5):599–604.

22. Vaidya R, Colen R, Vigdorchik J, et al. Treatment of unstable pelvic ring injuries with an internal anterior fixator and posterior fixation: initial clinical series. J Orthop Trauma 2012;26(1):1–8.

23. Vaidya R, Kubiak EN, Bergin PF, et al. Complications of anterior subcutaneous internal fixation for unstable pelvis fractures: a multicenter study. Clin Orthop Relat Res 2012;470(8):2124–31.

24. Porter SE, Graves ML, Qin Z, et al. Operative experience of pelvic fractures in the obese. Obes Surg 2008;18(6):702–8.

25. Sems SA, Johnson M, Cole PA, et al, Minnesota Orthopaedic Trauma Group. Elevated body mass index increases early complications of surgical treatment of pelvic ring injuries. J Orthop Trauma 2010;24(5):309–14.

26. Porter SE, Graves ML, Maples RA, et al. Acetabular fracture reductions in the obese patient. J Orthop Trauma 2011;25(6):371–7.

27. Mears DC, Velyvis JH, Chang CP. Displaced acetabular fractures managed operatively: indicators of outcome. Clin Orthop Relat Res 2003;(407): 173–86.

28. Porter SE, Russell GV, Dews RC, et al. Complications of acetabular fracture surgery in morbidly obese patients. J Orthop Trauma 2008;22(9):589–94.

29. Karunakar MA, Shah SN, Jerabek S. Body mass index as a predictor of complications after operative treatment of acetabular fractures. J Bone Joint Surg Am 2005;87(7):1498–502.

30. Sagi HC, Dziadosz D, Mir H, et al. Obesity, leukocytosis, embolization, and injury severity increase the risk for deep postoperative wound infection after pelvic and acetabular surgery. J Orthop Trauma 2013;27(1):6–10.

31. Morris BJ, Richards JE, Guillamondegui OD, et al. Obesity increases early complications after high-energy pelvic and acetabular fractures. Orthopedics 2015;38(10):e881–7.

32. Bergin PF, Kneip C, Pierce C, et al. Modifier 22 for acetabular fractures in morbidly obese patients: does it affect reimbursement? Clin Orthop Relat Res 2014;472(11):3370–4.

33. Reddix RN Jr, Tyler HK, Kulp B, et al. Incisional vacuum-assisted wound closure in morbidly obese patients undergoing acetabular fracture surgery. Am J Orthop (Belle Mead NJ) 2009;38(9):446–9.

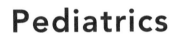

Pediatrics

The Musculoskeletal Aspects of Obesity in Neuromuscular Conditions

Michael J. Conklin, MD[a],*, Jeffrey M. Pearson, MD[b]

KEYWORDS

- Obesity • Spina bifida • Cerebral palsy • Muscular dystrophy • Musculoskeletal

---

KEY POINTS

- Obesity is extremely common in cerebral palsy, spina bifida, and Duchenne muscular dystrophy.
- Obesity in cerebral palsy can render computerized gait analysis less accurate.
- Obesity increases perioperative risks in neuromuscular patients, including an increased risk of infection after spinal instrumentation and fusion.
- Early dietary intervention and encouragement of physical activity through local health and wellness programs is imperative in controlling obesity in individuals with developmental disabilities.

OBESITY IN NEUROMUSCULAR CONDITIONS

Introduction

Obesity and overweight are epidemic among children in the United States.[1] The National Health and Nutrition Examination Survey (NHANES III) indicated that 14.4% of children and adolescents aged 2 to 19 years were overweight or obese.[2,3] A recent literature review revealed that the rate of obesity and overweight in children with disabilities was almost twice that of their nondisabled peers.[4] Furthermore, obesity is increasing in the United States and that increase is mirrored in patients with neuromuscular conditions. An investigation into the prevalence of obesity in ambulatory individuals with cerebral palsy (CP) disclosed an increase in the rate of obesity from 7.7% in the time period from 1994 to 1997 to 16.5% from 2003 to 2004.[5] Children with spina bifida have a 28% to 50% rate of obesity.[6–11] In addition to the typical health risks, obesity in individuals with neuromuscular disease can pose additional

challenges. Ambulation may be a laborious process for these individuals and the additional weight can affect this adversely.[12,13] Evaluation of these patients for possible orthopedic surgery can be made less accurate by obscuring of bony landmarks. Computerized gait analysis can be affected because of difficulties with marker ball placement[14,15] and the motion of marker balls because of abdominal pannus.[16] The performance of orthopedic procedures may be rendered more difficult and the complication rate may be higher because of obesity.[17,18] This article reviews the pertinent literature on the orthopedic aspects of obesity in individuals with neuromuscular conditions.

CEREBRAL PALSY

Introduction

CP is the leading cause of childhood disability,[19] and occurs in 2 to 2.5 per 1000 live births.[20] The rate of obesity is increasing in able-bodied children, and this is reflected in individuals with CP.[5,21] Hurvitz and colleagues[21] retrospectively

---

Disclosure: The authors have no disclosures.

[a] Department of Orthopedic Surgery, University of Cincinnati, UAB School of Medicine, Children's of Alabama, 1600 7th Avenue South, Lowder 316, Birmingham, AL 35233, USA; [b] Department of Orthopedic Surgery, Louisiana State University, UAB School of Medicine, Children's of Alabama, 1600 7th Avenue South, Lowder 316, Birmingham, AL 35233, USA
* Corresponding author.
E-mail address: mconklin@uabmc.edu

evaluated 137 children aged 2 to 18 years in a pediatric rehabilitation clinic. Body mass index (BMI) and Gross Motor Function Classification Score (GMFCS) were calculated and statistical analyses were performed. It was noted that 29.1% of children were considered overweight (>95th percentile) or at risk for overweight (85th–95th percentile). Ambulatory patients (GMFCS levels I and II) were more likely to be overweight than nonambulatory children (GMFCS levels IV and V). Underweight was more prevalent in nonambulatory children. In individuals with CP, the nonambulatory children are more likely to have feeding and swallowing dysfunction, which would confer on them a greater risk of underweight. A tendency for the more severely involved, nonambulatory children to be underweight has also been noted by other investigators.[22]

Multiple mechanisms may lead to overweight or obesity in children with CP. These children are often born premature or small for gestational age, both of which have been shown to be risk factors for obesity.[23–25] Body composition may be different in children with spastic quadriplegic CP, with a decrease in cell mass and expansion of the extracellular compartment.[26] Energy expenditure may be lower in these children and medical and social issues may restrict or preclude their participation in activities that are available to their able-bodied peers.[26–28] Risk of overweight in children and adolescents with CP are likely related to sedentary behavior. van den berg-Emons and colleagues[29] evaluated daily activity in 10 children with spastic diplegia and 10 children without disabilities. The children with CP were less active than their able-bodied peers, and the type of physical activity engaged in was not of an intensity that would be likely to improve their physical fitness. In addition, young people with spastic CP have been shown to have lower levels of aerobic capacity,[30,31] which may be partially caused by disruption of the reciprocal synchronization between agonist and antagonist muscle groups.[32]

Measurement

Measurement of BMI in individuals with CP and other disabilities may be problematic. Joint contractures, involuntary movements, and spinal deformity may render height or length measurement inaccurate.[20] Clinic personnel need to be adequately trained in measuring height in these individuals. Also, charts developed by the Centers for Disease Control and Prevention (www.cdc.gov) on BMI were developed for able-bodied individuals. Nevertheless, to date,

BMI is the most practical and easily reproducible method for expressing body composition.

The Effect of Obesity on Health and Function

Individuals with neuromuscular conditions and obesity have the same general health problems as obese individuals without neuromuscular problems. Obviously, this carries significant implications with regard to the risk of cardiovascular disease and diabetes in adulthood. Peterson and colleagues[33] found that, in adults with CP, abdominal obesity highly correlated with vitamin D deficiency.

In a study of neurologically normal children, fractures, musculoskeletal discomfort (particularly knee pain), impaired mobility, and lower extremity malalignment were more common in obese children.[34] It has been shown that neurologically normal children with obesity alter their gait to adapt to increased mass.[35,36] Obese children tend to collapse into hip adduction on the stance phase side, resulting in a Trendelenburg gait. This gait increases valgus stress at the knee, increasing the likelihood of future knee pain and arthritis.[37] The effect of obesity on function in ambulatory patients with CP is not completely understood. It is known that the sudden increase in weight during the adolescent growth spurt in diplegic CP is related to worsening crouch gait,[38] which may be caused by a declining strength/body mass ratio.[39] An increase in adipose tissue versus lean body mass would have an even more deleterious effect than the mere increase in size seen during the growth spurt.

Meyns and colleagues[12] experimentally evaluated the effect of increased weight on gait analysis parameters in children with CP and in typically developing children by adding 10% body weight using a belt around the waist. They noted that typically developing children increased their walking velocity, increased their step and stride length, and decreased their duration of double support, whereas the opposite pattern was found in CP. Typically developing children increased joint ranges of motion, angular velocities, moments, and powers, whereas CP children did not. In short, it seemed that CP children lacked the ability to compensate for experimentally added weight. With regard to nonambulatory patients, obesity can interfere with transfers and add to the burden of caretakers.

The Effect of Obesity on Patient Evaluation

Imperative to the orthopedic treatment of patients with CP is an accurate physical examination. Data on the accuracy of physical examination findings in obese individuals with neuromuscular conditions is lacking but information can be extrapolated from other studies. There may be some aspects of the physical examination that are rendered more difficult by obesity.[40] Bony landmarks such as the greater trochanter or malleoli used for evaluation of femoral anteversion or tibial torsion can be obscured by overlying subcutaneous fat. Although C-shaped curves with pelvic obliquity may be obvious, double major curves may be difficult to see until they are of moderate severity. In a study on patients with idiopathic scoliosis, a higher BMI correlated with greater curve magnitude on first presentation.[41]

Because of obesity, difficulties can be encountered in computerized gait analysis,[14,15] particularly in the placement of marker balls about the pelvis, because of difficulty identifying the anterior superior iliac spine and first sacral vertebra.[16] Furthermore, wobbling of subcutaneous fat can create soft tissue artifacts on gait analysis, making evaluation of anterior-posterior pelvic tilt less accurate.[16] In general, pelvic and transverse plane data may be less accurate in obese patients. Reliability can be improved by using different marker sets designed for obese patients.[14,42]

Effect of Obesity on Treatment
Nonsurgical
The effect of obesity on the orthopedic treatment of children and adolescents with CP can be divided into 2 categories: nonoperative and operative. One of the most common nonoperative treatments available to these patients is the use of braces, such as ankle foot orthoses. Obese patients are hard on their braces and normal wear and tear is accelerated, particularly about the ankle where bending or fatigue fractures of the brace are common. Strategies for boosting strength may include roping, double-layered polypropylene, or carbon fiber reinforcement.

Although data regarding the effectiveness of bracing scoliosis in CP and other neuromuscular conditions are lacking, it is often attempted in the hopes that surgery can be delayed or prevented. In patients with adolescent idiopathic scoliosis (AIS), literature suggests that overweight patients are 3.1 times less likely to have a successful result than those who are not overweight.[43] In another study on AIS, patients with BMI greater than the 85th percentile were noted to be more likely to fail treatment (as defined by curve progression) because of inadequacy of in-brace correction and poorer brace compliance.[44] Although specific studies regarding the effect of obesity on bracing in CP are lacking, the studies discussed earlier in AIS suggest that bracing would be less effective in obese individuals with CP. Future research on scoliosis bracing in this population is necessary.

Botulinum toxin injection may be used in the treatment of spastic muscles. Obesity may make palpating bony landmarks or reaching the muscle more difficult because of the increased thickness of the subcutaneous fat. An electromyography needle or ultrasonography guidance can be used to improve accuracy.[45] Extralong needles may be necessary to ensure that the injection is intramuscular.[46]

Surgical
Perioperative considerations. Obesity can render intubation more difficult and fiberoptic intubation is occasionally necessary.[47–50] In a study comparing obese and nonobese children undergoing dental procedures under general anesthesia, there was a higher risk of intraoperative oxygen desaturation and unplanned overnight hospitalization in the obese group.[51]

Surgical decision-making and performance may be altered in patients who are overweight or obese. Intraoperative positioning can be challenging and occasionally extralarge operating tables or bariatric bed extenders are necessary. Exposure is more laborious and fixation of osteotomies may need to be more robust because of greater anticipated forces. Postoperative mobilization may be more difficult for the patient, family, and physical therapist. Transfers are harder on the caretakers and can result in a greater risk of mishaps. Increased weight and obesity restricts movement and may negatively affect the ability to rehabilitate after gait corrective surgery.[52,53]

Some complications occur with higher frequency in obese patients. Ishola and colleagues[54] noted obesity to be a risk factor in adolescent thromboembolism. Obesity has been shown to increase the risk of infection after spine surgery for neuromuscular scoliosis. In a retrospective study of patients undergoing posterior spinal fusion (PSF) for neuromuscular scoliosis, BMI greater than 25 kg/m^2 correlated with an increased risk of surgical site infection.[17] Another study evaluating complications of PSF in neuromuscular scoliosis showed that infectious complications were associated with a BMI greater than or equal to the 95th percentile.[18]

MYELOMENINGOCELE

Introduction

The rate of obesity ranges from 28% to 50% in children and 34% to 64% in adults with spina bifida.[1-11] Most children with spina bifida follow a typical growth pattern until 4 years of age and then start to diverge from their able-bodied peers, developing increased fat mass versus lean mass.[55,56] Thereafter, the rate of obesity increases with age across the lifespan.[6,57]

Individuals with developmental disabilities are at risk for lower rates of regular physical activity.[58] Causes of obesity in spina bifida may include nonambulatory status, sedentary lifestyle, neuroendocrine disturbances, differences in body composition, and lower basal metabolic rates.[7,8,10,11] There are many barriers to physical activity for these individuals, including transportation, cost of adaptive equipment, and lack of adaptive physical education in the schools.[6,59,60] Medical comorbidities such as shunted hydrocephalus, incontinence, and skin breakdown can limit participation in physical activity.[6] In addition, patients may be temporarily limited in their ability to participate in activities because of restrictions after orthopedic surgery.

Measurement

Obesity rates among people with spina bifida have been assessed by a variety of methods.[7-11,55-57] BMI is an imperfect indicator of health in spina bifida.[61] Individuals with spina bifida may not have the same anthropometric characteristics as able-bodied individuals and may have a short trunk,[7,57,62] particularly those with higher levels of neurologic lesions, and these differences can be exacerbated by spinal deformity.[62] For this reason, arm span has been used as a proxy for height when calculating BMI.[9,62]

Effect on Health and Function

Individuals with spina bifida and obesity have an increased risk of various health problems, including decubitus ulcers, gastroesophageal reflux disease, metabolic syndrome, depression, and reduced mobility and independence.[63,64] Nelson and colleagues, evaluated the frequency of metabolic syndrome in adolescents with spinal cord injury and spina bifida. They noted that metabolic syndrome was present in 45.8% of patients with spina bifida and 100% of patients with spinal cord injury.[63] Obesity has been shown to adversely affect ambulation and has been shown to be a factor in transitioning to a lower ambulatory status.[13] Individuals with spina bifida can develop lower extremity physeal

stress fractures and Charcot changes so it is concerning that increased weight further stresses the bones, joints, and tendons (**Fig. 1**). Children with spina bifida are at increased risk of fractures, especially those who are nonambulatory and have low levels of physical activity and higher body fat.[65]

Effect on Treatment

Individuals with spina bifida and obesity can pose a challenge for orthopedic surgeons, particularly for midlumbar-level adolescents who are spending less time ambulating and have musculoskeletal deformities in need of correction. In these cases, candid conversations need to occur between the patient, family, and surgeon regarding the surgical risks and arduous rehabilitation process. Fixation of osteotomies may need to be more robust than usual in order to allow early mobilization and weight bearing. In spite of this, periprosthetic fractures occur with increased frequency in spina bifida because of osteopenia and, although data are lacking, likely occur with higher frequency in those who are obese. As previously discussed, infection rates after spine surgery in neuromuscular scoliosis are increased in patients who are obese.[17,18] Perioperative antibiotics should include gram-negative coverage.

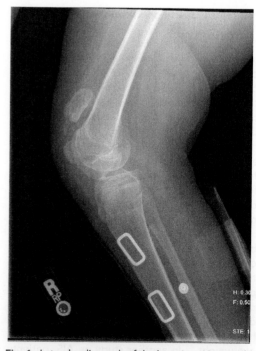

Fig. 1. Lateral radiograph of the knee in a 12-year-old obese girl with midlumbar-level myelomeningocele with crouch gait complaining of knee pain. Note the patellar fragmentation.

The most important treatment of obesity in spina bifida is prevention. Dietary intervention should begin early and patients should be encouraged to participate in physical activity.[59,66,67] Community-based health and wellness programs and venues for individuals with disability are extremely helpful. Rimmer and colleagues[68] describe a framework for building and maintaining a database of successful health and wellness guidelines to promote community inclusion for people with disabilities.

Duchenne Muscular Dystrophy

Duchenne muscular dystrophy (DMD) is the second most common hereditary genetic disease in humans, with X-linked inheritance. Corticosteroids are now a mainstay of treatment of this condition and various regimens have been proposed.[69–71] Corticosteroids can help to preserve muscle strength, prolong ambulation, reduce the need for scoliosis surgery, improve pulmonary function, delay cardiomyopathy, and improve survival.[69–71] Long-term side effects of corticosteroids include obesity, decreased bone mineral density, and reduction in vitamin D levels.[70,72] There is debate as to whether decreased resting energy expenditure plays a role in the development of obesity in these boys.[73] Nevertheless, it is clear that body composition is altered in DMD because of fatty infiltration of muscles and therefore special techniques such as bioelectrical impedance analysis may be necessary to accurately assess obesity.[74] A more simple approach is to use reference charts developed by Griffiths and Edwards[75] for body weight/age ratio. Early detection of fat accumulation may allow dietary intervention, which may help to lessen the burden that obesity adds to DMD. These boys may go through an evolution with regard to body composition such that obesity is most common in the early teens, whereas a large percentage of patients in their late teens or early adulthood are underweight.[76] One study noted that 73% of boys were obese at 13 years of age, whereas another noted that 50% were obese at 10 years of age.[76,77] It seems that patients with DMD who are obese in the early teens are most likely to remain obese, whereas those who are normal weight or underweight at that time are at risk for underweight later.[76] This trend could be caused by higher energy expenditure as these individuals start to experience respiratory failure.[78]

Individuals with DMD may experience the same metabolic complications of obesity as their able-bodied peers, such as insulin resistance and dyslipidemia.[79] Nevertheless, there is a paucity of literature specifically addressing the musculoskeletal complications of obesity in this population. Although it is known that the age at which most of these boys are obese is also the age at which they abandon ambulation, it is hard to prove a causal relationship. One study noted that those who had lost ambulation had a significantly higher percentage of fat mass than those in whom ambulation was preserved.[79]

Approximately 25% of patients with DMD experience a long bone fracture. One nuance worth pointing out, because of the significant morbidity or mortality involved, is that individuals with DMD may develop fat embolism syndrome from minor fractures.[80,81] This syndrome may be difficult to recognize because of preexisting pulmonary issues so a high index of suspicion should be maintained.

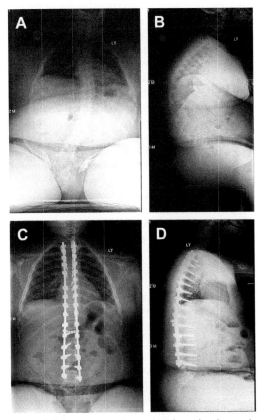

Fig. 2. (A) Anteroposterior and (B) lateral radiographs of the spine in an obese 13-year-old boy with Duchenne and spinal deformity interfering with sitting balance. (C, D) Patient underwent posterior spinal fusion and instrumentation complicated by deep wound infection with *Escherichia coli*. This infection required multiple irrigations and debridements and intravenous antibiotics.

Lower extremity soft tissue surgery can help to delay the loss of ambulation.[82] Care must be taken to mobilize quickly and avoid weight gain after surgery, which can compromise the ambulatory status.[82]

Scoliosis is a common occurrence in DMD, particularly after ambulation is lost, and the natural history is one of progression. If spinal deformity surgery is contemplated, it should be noted that obesity increases the risk of infection after spine surgery for neuromuscular scoliosis[17,18] (Fig. 2).

SUMMARY

Obesity is a common problem in neuromuscular conditions. In ambulatory patients, it can negatively affect ambulation, worsen crouch gait, and increase stress on musculoskeletal structures. In nonambulators, obesity makes transfers more difficult and increases the burden on caretakers. Physical examination may be less accurate and deformities such as scoliosis may be seen later, when they are of a greater magnitude. Computerized gait analysis can be more challenging because of inaccuracy of marker ball placement and abdominal pannus. Nonoperative treatments, such as botulinum toxin injection and bracing, may be more difficult. Surgical treatment carries increased morbidity, such as an increased rate of thromboembolism and infection. Treatment should be aimed at prevention, with an eye toward early dietary modification and increased physical activity. On a societal level, efforts should be made to improve/increase adaptive physical education and facilities in the community that allow for the inclusion of individuals with disabilities in physical activities.

REFERENCES

1. Strauss RS, Pollack HA. Epidemic increase in childhood overweight, 1986-1998. JAMA 2001;286: 2845–8.
2. Ogden CL, Flegal KM, Carroll MD, et al. Prevalence and trends in overweight among US children and adolescents, 1999-2000. JAMA 2002;288:1728–32.
3. Troiano RP, Flegal KM. Overweight children and adolescents: description, epidemiology, and demographics. Pediatrics 1998;101:497–504.
4. Reinehr T, Dobe M, Winkel K, et al. Obesity in disabled children and adolescents: an overlooked group of patients. Dtsch Arztebl Int 2010;107: 268–75.
5. Rogozinski BM, Davids JR, Davis RB, et al. Prevalence of obesity in ambulatory children with cerebral palsy. J Bone Joint Surg Am 2007;89:2421–6.
6. Dosa NP, Foley JT, Eckrich M, et al. Obesity across the lifespan among persons with spina bifida. Disabil Rehabil 2009;31:914–20.
7. Hayes-Allen MC. Obesity and short stature in children with myelomeningocele. Dev Med Child Neurol Suppl 1972;27:59–64.
8. Mita K, Akataki K, Itoh K, et al. Assessment of obesity of children with spina bifida. Dev Med Child Neurol 1993;35:305–11.
9. Jarzem PF, Gledhill RB. Predicting height from arm measurements. J Pediatr Orthop 1993;13:761–5.
10. Van den Berg-Emons HJ, Bussmann JB, Meyerink HJ, et al. Body fat, fitness and level of everyday physical activity in adolescents and young adults with meningomyelocele. J Rehabil Med 2003;35:271–5.
11. Roebroeck ME, Hempenius L, VanBaalen B, et al. Cognitive functioning of adolescents and young adults with meningomyelocele and level of everyday physical activity. Disabil Rehabil 2006;28: 1237–42.
12. Meyns P, Van Gestel L, Bar-On L, et al. Children with spastic cerebral palsy experience difficulties adjusting their gait pattern to weight added to the waist, while typically developing children do not. Front Hum Neurosci 2016;10:657.
13. Asher M, Olson J. Factors affecting the ambulatory status of patients with spina bifida cystica. J Bone Joint Surg Am 1983;65(3):350–6.
14. Lerner ZF, Board WJ, Browning RC. Effects of an obesity-specific marker set on estimated muscle and joint forces in walking. Med Sci Sports Exerc 2014;46:1261–7.
15. Peters A, Galna B, Sangeux M, et al. Quantification of soft tissue artifact in lower limb human motion analysis: a systematic review. Gait Posture 2010; 31:1–8.
16. Horsak B, Schwab C, Clemens C, et al. Is the reliability of 3D kinematics of young obese participants dependent on the hip joint center localization method used? Gait Posture 2017;59:65–70.
17. Ramo BA, Roberts DW, Tuason D, et al. Surgical site infections after posterior spinal fusion for neuromuscular scoliosis. J Bone Joint Surg Am 2014;96:2038–48.
18. Basques BA, Chung SH, Lukasiewicz AM, et al. Predicting short-term morbidity in patients undergoing posterior spinal fusion for neuromuscular scoliosis. Spine (Phila Pa 1976) 2015;40(24):1910–7.
19. Stanley F. Cerebral palsy trends: implications for perinatal care. Acta Obstet Gynecol Scand 1994; 73:5–9.
20. Nelson KB, Ellenberg JH. Epidemiology of cerebral palsy. Adv Neurol 1978;19:421–35.
21. Hurvitz EA, Green LB, Hornyak JE, et al. Body mass index measures in children with cerebral palsy related to gross motor function classification: a

clinic-based study. Am J Phys Med Rehabil 2008;87: 395–403.

22. Simsek TT, Tuc G. Examination of the relation between body mass index, functional level and health-related quality of life in children with cerebral palsy. Turk Pediatri Ars 2014;49:130–7.

23. Hales CN, Barker DJ. The thrifty phenotype hypothesis. Br Med Bull 2002;60:5–20.

24. Hales CN, Barker DJ, Clark PM, et al. Fetal and infant growth and impaired glucose tolerance at age 64. BMJ 1991;303:1010–22.

25. Curhan GC, Chertow GM, Willett WC, et al. Birth weight and adult hypertension and obesity in women. Circulation 1996;94:1310–5.

26. Bandini LG, Schoeller DA, Fukagawa NK, et al. Body composition and energy expenditure in adolescents with cerebral palsy or myelodysplasia. Pediatr Res 1991;29:70–7.

27. Stallings VA, Cronk CE, Zemel BS, et al. Body composition in children with spastic quadriplegic cerebral palsy. J Pediatr 1995;126:833–9.

28. Azcue MP, Zello GA, Levy LD, et al. Energy expenditure and body composition in children with spastic quadriplegic cerebral palsy. J Pediatr 1996;129: 870–6.

29. van den Berg-Emons HJ, Saris WH, de Barbanson DC, et al. Daily physical activity of schoolchildren with spastic diplegia and of healthy control subjects. J Pediatr 1995;127:578–84.

30. Lundberg A. Maximal aerobic capacity of young people with spastic cerebral palsy. Dev Med Child Neurol 1978;20:205–10.

31. Lundberg A. Longitudinal study of physical working capacity of young people with spastic cerebral palsy. Dev Med Child Neurol 1984;26:328–34.

32. Parker DF, Carriere L, Hebestreit H, et al. Anaerobic endurance and peak muscle power in children with spastic cerebral palsy. Am J Dis Child 1993;146: 1069–73.

33. Peterson MD, Haapala H, Chaddha A, et al. Abdominal obesity is an independent predictor of serum 25-hydroxyvitamin D deficiency in adults with cerebral palsy. Nutr Metab (Lond) 2014;11:22.

34. Taylor ED, Theim KR, Mirch MC, et al. Orthopedic complications of overweight in children and adolescents. Pediatrics 2006;117(6):2167–74.

35. Blakemore VJ, Fink PW, Lark SD, et al. Mass affects lower extremity muscle activity patterns in children's gait. Gait Posture 2013;38(4):609–13.

36. de Sá Pinto AL, de Barros Holanda PM, Radu AS, et al. Musculoskeletal findings in obese children. J Paediatr Child Health 2006;42(6):341–4.

37. Shultz SP, D'Hondt E, Fink PW, et al. The effects of pediatric obesity on dynamic joint malalignment during gait. Clin Biomech (Bristol, Avon) 2014; 29(7):835–8.

38. Gage JR. Treatment principles for crouch gait. In: Gage JR, editor. Treatment of gait problems in cerebral palsy. London: Mac Keith Press; 2004. p. 382–97.

39. Kedem P, Scher DM. Evaluation and management of crouch gait. Curr Opin Pediatr 2016;28:55–9.

40. Silk AW, McTigue KM. Reexamining the physical examination for obese patients. JAMA 2011; 305(2):193–4.

41. Gilbert SR, Conklin MJ, Savage AJ, et al. BMI and magnitude of scoliosis at presentation to a specialty clinic. Pediatrics 2015;135(6):e1417–24.

42. Borhani M, McGregor MH, Bull AMJ. An alternative technical marker set for the pelvis is more repeatable than the standard pelvic marker set. Gait Posture 2013;38:1032–7.

43. O'Neill PJ, Karol LA, Shindle MK, et al. Decreased orthotic effectiveness in overweight patients with adolescent idiopathic scoliosis. J Bone Joint Surg Am 2005;87(5):1069–73.

44. Goodbody CM, Sankar WN, Flynn JM. Presentation of adolescent idiopathic scoliosis: the bigger the kid, the bigger the curve. J Pediatr Orthop 2017; 37:41–6.

45. Py AG, Zein AG, Perrier Y, et al. Evaluation of the effectiveness of botulinum toxin injections in the lower limb muscles of children with cerebral palsy. Preliminary prospective study of the advantages of ultrasound guidance. Ann Phys Rehabil Med 2009; 52(3):215–23.

46. Zaybak A, Gunes UY, Tamsel S, et al. Does obesity prevent the needle from reaching muscle in intramuscular injections? J Adv Nurs 2007;58(6): 552–6.

47. Sabharwal S, Root MZ. Impact of obesity on orthopaedics. J Bone Joint Surg Am 2012;94:1045–52.

48. Juvin P, Lavaut E, Dupont H, et al. Difficult tracheal intubation is more common in obese than in lean patients. Anesth Analg 2003;97(2):595–600.

49. Lundstrøm LH, Møller AM, Rosenstock C, et al. High body mass index is a weak predictor for difficult and failed tracheal intubation: a cohort study of 91,332 consecutive patients scheduled for direct laryngoscopy registered in the Danish anesthesia database. Anesthesiology 2009;110(2):266–74.

50. Fujinaga A, Fukushima Y, Kojima A, et al. Anesthetic management of an extremely obese patient. J Anesth 2007;21(2):261–4.

51. Setzer N, Saade E. Childhood obesity and anesthetic morbidity. Paediatr Anaesth 2007;17(4): 321–6.

52. Padwal RS, Wang X, Sharma AM, et al. The impact of severe obesity on post-acute rehabilitation efficiency, length of stay, and hospital costs. J Obes 2012;2012:972365.

53. Pascoe J, Thomason P, Graham HK, et al. Body mass index in ambulatory children with cerebral

palsy: a cohort study. J Paediatr Child Health 2016; 52:417–21.

54. Ishola T, Kirk SE, Guffey D, et al. Risk factors and co-morbidities in adolescent thromboembolism are different than those in younger children. Thromb Res 2016;141:178–82.

55. Shepherd K, Roberts D, Golding S, et al. Body composition in myelomeningocele. Am J Clin Nutr 1991;53:1–6.

56. Littlewood R, Trocku O, Shepherd R, et al. Resting energy expenditure and body composition in children with myelomeningocele. Pediatr Rehabil 2003;6:31–7.

57. Roberts D, Shepherd RW, Shepherd K. Anthropometry and obesity in myelomeningocele. J Paediatr Child Health 1991;27:83–90.

58. US Department of Health and Human Services. Healthy people 2010, 2nd edition. With understanding and improving health and objectives for improving health, vol. 2. Washington, DC: US Government Printing Office; 2000.

59. An J, Goodwin DL. Physical education for children with spina bifida: a mother's perspective. Adapt Phys Activ Q 2007;24:38–58.

60. Rimmer JH, Rowland JL, Yamaki K. Obesity and secondary conditions in adolescents with disabilities: addressing the needs of an underserved population. J Adolesc Health 2007;41: 224–9.

61. Polfuss M, Simpson P, Stolzman S, et al. The measurement of body composition in children with spina bifida: Feasibility and preliminary findings. J Pediatr Rehabil Med 2016;9:143–53.

62. Rosenblum MF, Finegold DN, Charney EB. Assessment of stature of children with myelomeningocele, and usefulness of arm-span measurement. Dev Med Child Neurol 1983;25:338–42.

63. Nelson MD, Widman LM, Abresch RT, et al. Metabolic syndrome in adolescents with spinal cord dysfunction. J Spinal Cord Med 2007;30: S127–39.

64. Simeonsson RJ, McMillen JS, Huntington GS. Secondary conditions in children with disabilities: spina bifida as a case example. Ment Retard Dev Disabil Res Rev 2002;8:198–205.

65. Marreiros H, Loff C, Calado E. Osteoporosis in paediatric patients with spina bifida. J Spinal Cord Med 2012;35:9–21.

66. Grogan CB, Ekvall SM. Body composition of children with myelomeningocele, determined by 40K, urinary creatinine and anthropometric measures. J Am Coll Nutr 1999;18:316–23.

67. Schultz AW, Liptak GS. Obesity, insights factsheet, Spina Bifida Association of America. Internet. Available at: http://www.sbaa.org/site/c.liKWL7PLLrF/b.2700287/k.C25F/Obesity.htm. Assessed November 29, 2007.

68. Rimmer JH, Vanderbom KA, Graham ID. A new framework and practice center for adapting, translating, and scaling evidence-based health/wellness programs for people with disabilities. J Neurol Phys Ther 2016;40(2):107–14.

69. Connolly AM, Schierbeck J, Renna R, et al. High dose weekly oral prednisone improves strength in boys with Duchenne muscular dystrophy. Neuromuscul Disord 2002;12(10):917–25.

70. Pradhan S, Ghosh D, Srivastava NK, et al. Prednisolone in Duchenne muscular dystrophy with imminent loss of ambulation. J Neurol 2006;253(10): 1309–16.

71. Gloss D, Moxley RT, Ashwal S, et al. Practice guideline update summary: corticosteroid treatment of Duchenne muscular dystrophy: report of the Guideline Development Subcommittee of the American Academy of Neurology. Neurology 2016;86(5):465–72.

72. Jeronimo G, Nozoe KT, Polesel DN, et al. Impact of corticotherapy, nutrition, and sleep disorder on quality of life of patients with Duchenne muscular dystrophy. Nutrition 2016;32(3):391–3.

73. Zanardi MC, Tagliabue A, Orcesi S, et al. Body composition and energy expenditure in Duchenne muscular dystrophy. Eur J Clin Nutr 2003;57(2): 273–8.

74. Mok E, Beghin L, Gachon P, et al. Estimating body composition in children with Duchenne muscular dystrophy: comparison of bioelectrical impedance analysis and skinfold-thickness measurement. Am J Clin Nutr 2006;83(1):65–9.

75. Griffiths RD, Edwards RH. A new chart for weight control in Duchenne muscular dystrophy. Arch Dis Child 1988;63(10):1256–8.

76. Martigne L, Sallerson J, Mayer M, et al. Natural evolution of weight status in Duchenne muscular dystrophy: a retrospective audit. Br J Nutr 2011; 105(10):1486–91.

77. Davidson ZE, Ryan MM, Kornberg AJ, et al. Observations of body mass index in Duchenne muscular dystrophy: a longitudinal study. Eur J Clin Nutr 2014;68(8):892–7.

78. Shimizu-Fujiwara M, Komaki H, Nakagawa E, et al. Decreased resting energy expenditure in patients with Duchenne muscular dystrophy. Brain Dev 2012;34(3):206–12.

79. Saure C, Caminiti C, Weglinski J, et al. Energy expenditure, body composition, and prevalence of metabolic disorders in patients with Duchenne muscular dystrophy. Diabetes Metab Syndr 2017 [pii:S1871-4021(17)30276-X].

80. Feder D, Koch ME, Palmiere B, et al. Fat embolism after fractures in Duchenne muscular dystrophy: an underdiagnosed complication? A systematic review. Ther Clin Risk Manag 2017; 13:1357–61.

81. Stein L, Herold R, Austin A, et al. Fat emboli syndrome in a child with Duchenne muscular dystrophy after minor trauma. J Emerg Med 2016;50(5): e223–6.

82. Smith SE, Green NE, Cole RJ, et al. Prolongation of ambulation in children with Duchenne muscular dystrophy by subcutaneous lower limb tenotomy. J Pediatr Orthop 1993;13:336–40.

83. Hollander SA, Rizzuto S, Hollander AM, et al. Obesity and premature loss of mobility in two adolescents with Becker muscular dystrophy after heartmate II implantation. ASAIO J 2016;62(1):e5–7.

Obesity in Pediatric Trauma

Philip Ashley, MD, Shawn R. Gilbert, MD*

KEYWORDS

- Obesity • Pediatric • Trauma • Fracture

KEY POINTS

- Compared to non-obese children, obese children with high-energy injuries present with more severe injuries, more extremity injuries, and higher Injury Severity Scores. They are at increased risk for complications, prolonged ventilation, and ICU stay and have increased mortality.
- Obesity is associated with altered bone mass accrual and higher fracture rates.
- Obese patients have a higher risk of loss of reduction of forearm fractures, more severe supracondylar fractures, and a higher likelihood of lateral condyle fractures.
- Obese patients are more likely to have complications with femur fractures and have higher rates of foot and ankle fracture.
- Special considerations may be needed for cast management, surgical positioning, implant choice, and infection prevention.

INTRODUCTION

This review presents updates on the occurrence and management of orthopedic injuries in obese pediatric patients, including polytrauma patients (high-energy trauma that typically results in a trauma alert and/or results in injuries to multiple organ systems). Unless otherwise specified, all studies discussed and referenced specifically examine pediatric patients. Differences in injury risk, injury patterns, and management are discussed. Outcomes of treatments, including increased risk of complications, are reviewed. Strategies to manage obese patients appropriately and avoid complications are also discussed.

THE OBESE PEDIATRIC POLYTRAUMA PATIENT

Susceptibility to Polytrauma Injury

Both obesity and polytrauma are major public health concerns. Overall, rates of trauma admissions seem similar between obese and nonobese patients, but studies have found conflicting results regarding possible differences in injury patterns, severity, and outcomes.[1-5] Some studies have found that obese pediatric patents present with higher Injury Severity Score (ISS),[2,5] whereas others (including the 2 largest studies) found no difference in ISS.[3] There may be differences with respect to injury patterns, however. A study using data from 149,817 patients in the 2013 to 2014 National Trauma Data Bank data sets found that higher body mass index (BMI) percentiles were associated with more extremity injuries and fewer and less severe injuries to the head, thorax, abdomen, and spine.[1] Other studies also found that injury patterns may differ in that obese pediatric patients are more likely to have solid organ injury and hollow viscus injury[5] and experience more severe solid organ injury.[6] Additionally, with respect to skeletal injury, obese pediatric patients were more likely to have pelvic fractures[2,5] and more likely to present with bilateral tibia fractures.[5] Findings related to these studies are summarized in **Table 1**.

Disclosure Statement: No relevant financial interests.
Department of Orthopaedic Surgery, University of Alabama Birmingham, 1600 7th Avenue South, Lowder 316, Birmingham, AL 35233, USA
* Corresponding author.
E-mail address: srgilbert@uabmc.edu

Orthop Clin N Am 49 (2018) 335–343
https://doi.org/10.1016/j.ocl.2018.02.007

Table 1
Summary of studies examining obesity in polytrauma

Study Period (Reference)	Inclusion	Setting	Number of Patients	Effect of Obesity on Severity	Effect of Obesity on Injury Patterns	Effect of Obesity on Outcomes
1998–2003 (Brown et al,[4] 2006)	Trauma admissions to ICU	ICU single center (US)	316	Less severe head injuries	No difference	↑Complication ↑ICU stay
2001–9 (Alselaim et al,[2] 2012)	All trauma	Single-center trauma registry (Saudi Arabia)	933 (75% excluded—no height/weight)	Obesity: ↑ISS ↓Peds trauma score	↑Pelvic fractures Slight ↑extremity injuries	No difference mortality
2004–7 (Rana et al,[3] 2009)	All trauma	Single center (US)	1314 (73% of database missing height or weight)	No difference	↑ Extremity injuries ↓Abdominal, head injuries	↑Surgery extremities ↑Decubitus ↑DVT
2004–10 (Backstrom et al,[5] 2012)	All trauma with Lower extremity fracture	Trauma registry 2 centers (US)	356 (16.6% no height, used WFA, not BMI)	↑ISS ↑ICU admission	↑Abdominal ↑Pelvic fracture ↑Bilateral tibia	↑ Mortality (RR 3.45, no effect when adjusted for age, ISS) ↑Femur operative fixation ↑LOS
2013–2014 (Witt et al,[1] 2017)	All trauma (exclude isolated burns)	National Trauma Data Bank (US)	149,817 (30% missing height—imputed)	No difference	↑Extremity injuries ↓Head, thorax, abdomen, spine injuries	↑Mortality (RR 1.11) ↑Any complication (RR 1.13) ↑DVT/PE (0.2%→0.3%) ↑LOS

Abbreviations: PE, pulmonary embolus; peds, pediatric; WFA, weight for age.

Many of the studies rely on databases that are frequently missing accurate height or weight measurements, requiring excluding large numbers of patients or making statistical adjustments. The authors suggest stressing recording accurate height and weight measurements wherever possible both to monitor patients' changes over time and possibly for inclusion in future research.

Although differences in fracture patterns are not well understood, computer modeling has demonstrated that head and trunk excursion and head injury and chest acceleration correlated with BMI increase in restrained computational 3-year-old and 6-year-old patient models, suggesting that increased BMI could increase risk of injury or severity of injury to the head and chest.[7] Additional speculation includes impaired fit of restraints or increased likelihood of improper restraint application.

Polytrauma is associated with systemic responses, and these may be altered in obese patients. Although adipokines are believed associated with inflammation, the effects of obesity on the systemic response to injury are not clear. In obese polytrauma patients, some studies suggest increased mortality[1,5] as well as longer ICU stays.[4,5] In contrast, differences in ventilator days, complications, or mortality are not seen in the general pediatric ICU population[8] or a pediatric burn population.[9]

Some differences in complication rates have also been found in pediatric trauma patients. When multivariate analysis was performed in the National Trauma Data Bank study, using BMI as a continuous variable, there were significant increases in the relative risk of deep venous thrombosis (DVT) and pulmonary embolism.[1] This was also found in a single-center study.[3] Although in both studies, the rate of DVT was still less than 1%, it points to the need for increased vigilance in obese patients, who may experience more stasis from increased difficulty mobilizing. Other complications noted at higher rates included decubitus ulcers[3] and any complication.[1,4]

With possibly more severe presentation and higher complication rates, higher health care utilization could be expected. Several studies showed increased LOS overall and longer ICU length of stay (LOS)[1,4,5] as well as higher rates of surgical intervention for extremity injuries[3,5] (although a smaller single-center study showed no difference in LOS or utilization of resources[10]). A study specifically examining cost found that obese patients admitted with fracture or dislocation had significantly higher median charges than nonobese patients.[11]

FRACTURE RISK IN OBESE PATIENTS

Obesity is associated with increased bone mass and increased bone mineral density (BMD) in children and adolescents.[12,13] This is presumed due to the effects of Wolff's law whereby increased weight bearing promotes bone deposition. The relationship is likely not that simple: for example, increased abdominal fat thickness is negatively correlated with BMD in obese children and adolescents.[14] Concerns also exist regarding the quality of the bone and its strength. More precise studies using peripheral quantitative CT, which allows for evaluating not only bone density but also bone architecture, raise concerns about the volumetric density of bone and highlight that there may also be differences between upper and lower extremities.[12,15] In addition to the mechanical effects of obesity, there are differences in onset of puberty, trends towards vitamin D deficiency (possibly due to sequestration of this fat-soluble hormone), and direct effects of adipokines such as leptin (reviewed by Dimitri and colleagues[16]). Bone health guidelines from the American Academy of Pediatrics note the associations with low BMD and underweight as well as potential negative effects of adiposity with fracture risk and recommend maintenance of healthy body weight and weight-bearing exercise.[17]

Regardless of possible increases in BMD, pediatric obesity is associated with increased fracture rate. A case-control study of patients presenting to outpatient clinics with fractures found that in girls with fractures, obesity was more common than in girls in the control group. In boys, however, obesity was only increased in those with lower extremity fractures.[18] Similarly, forearm fractures from ground-level falls are more likely to occur in patients with increased weight status.[19] Two studies examined associations between obesity and musculoskeletal complaints using the Kaiser Permanente Southern California Children's Health Study, which included 913,178 patients over a 3-year period in a large population-based cohort study. In the first study, Adams and colleagues[20] demonstrated increased risk of lower extremity fracture (as well as musculoskeletal pain complaints, sprains, and dislocations) in overweight and obese children compared with normal-weight children. In a follow-up study, Kessler and colleagues[21] examined the association between weight status and lower extremity fracture sites. Overweight and obesity were associated with increased odds of fractures of the foot, ankle, leg, and knee. These were most pronounced in the 6-year-old to 11-year-old age group. There was no association between obesity and fracture risk for the femur and hip.[21] These studies contribute to the body of evidence suggesting that obesity is associated with fracture risk early in childhood, but as patients reach adolescence, fractures are more often associated with sports activities (which are less commonly undertaken by obese patients[22]) and the increased fracture risk is diminished by decreased exposure to at risk activities.

Fracture Patterns

When fractures do occur, it might be suspected that the increased mass associated with obesity would result in increased force applied to the skeleton and, consequently, more severe fractures. This has not turned out to be the case in general. Fractures in obese patients presenting to an emergency department were not more likely to be severe (open fracture or those requiring reduction or surgery).[23] There may be some generalizable differences in fracture patterns, including an increased rate of physeal fractures in lower extremities.[24]

UPPER EXTREMITY FRACTURES

Forearm Fractures

Forearm fractures are the most common pediatric fracture and account for significant health care expenditure and potential morbidity.

Rana and colleagues[3] evaluated 1314 patients and found that obese patients had a significantly higher incidence of extremity fractures (55% vs 40%; P<.001). They also noted that the obese patients tended to receive operative treatment of their extremity fractures at a greater rate (42% vs 30%; P<.001). The location of extremity injuries was not further clarified in the study. The following year, Pomerantz and colleagues[25] reviewed 23,349 patients who had documented weights found no difference in the incidence of upper extremity injuries (36.3% vs 36.3%) but did note that obese children were more likely to suffer lower extremity injuries (29.8% vs 17.5%; odds ratio [OR] 1.85–2.17). Only 5% of the patients in this study group were admitted to the hospital and a significant portion of the lower extremity injuries were found to be sprains. In addition, the obesity status was calculated based on a patient's weight and age without any documented height measurements.

To further elucidate the effect of weight on low-energy forearm fractures, Ryan and colleagues[26] performed a retrospective case-control study of 280 patients (226 low energy vs 54 major trauma). They found that the ground-level fall fracture patients were older (10.4 vs 7.4; P<.5) and more likely to be obese (OR 2.7; 95% CI, 1.2–6.5).[10] Using an expanded group of 853 patients from this same data set, Ryan and colleagues also compared those who underwent reduction (n = 326) and those who did not require reduction (n = 527) and found no difference in the incidence of obesity between the 2 groups.[26]

Recent studies regarding obesity and forearm fractures have focused on treatment implications of obesity. Hirsch and colleagues[27] examined the rates of oxygen desaturation during procedural sedation for manipulative reduction of long bone fractures. In a retrospective review of 814 patients, they found obese children had greater desaturation rates (9.9% vs 5.4%; P = .035). Further analysis of this discrepancy identified that this difference disappeared when patients were dosed for their sedation by ideal body weight. Three recent studies have also highlighted the difficulties encountered when attempting to treat pediatric forearm fractures through closed means. Auer and colleagues[28] reviewed 157 consecutive distal radius fractures and found that obese children were more likely to require a second reduction (28% vs 12%; P = .02). DeFrancesco and colleagues[29] and Okoroafor and colleagues[30] published similar studies both showing that obese patients with diaphyseal both bone forearm fractures are more likely to experience a loss of reduction during the course of cast treatment (44.4% vs 7.2%; P = .005 and 34% vs 18%; P = .04, respectively). These studies also found nonsignificant trends toward surgical management among the obese patients after the initial failure of nonoperative treatment.

These published data seem to indicate that pediatric forearm fractures are more likely to occur in the obese population and especially in the setting of high-energy trauma. Caring for these patients requires vigilance in the acute setting to ensure appropriate reduction as well as an increased vigilance of the sedation team to dose the sedation medications by ideal body weight and be alert for and promptly intervene when desaturation occurs. After initial reduction is obtained, obese patients have a high propensity to lose reduction and require further intervention. For this reason, the authors recommend frequent radiographic observation of obese patients to identify and intervene appropriately when loss of reduction does occur.

Elbow Fractures

Obesity has also been implicated with an increasing risk for fractures of the distal humerus. Fornari and colleagues[31] reviewed 992 patients with fractures of the distal humerus and found that those with lateral condyle fractures were more likely to be obese than those with supracondylar humerus fractures (37% vs 19%; $P<.001$). Within the lateral condyle group (n = 230), there was also a higher percentage of obese patients with type 3 fractures than with type 2 or type 1 fractures (44% vs 27% and 26%, respectively; $P = .05$). A similar subgroup analysis of the supracondylar humerus fracture group did not find any association between fracture classification and obesity.

In 2014, Seeley and colleagues[32] published a review of 354 supracondylar humerus fractures treated at a single institution. Using a logistic regression analysis, they found associated with complex fractures (OR 9.19; $P<.001$), preoperative nerve palsies (OR 2.69; $P = .02$), postoperative nerve palsies (OR 7.69; $P<.001$), and postoperative complications (OR 4.03; $P<.001$). Sangkomkamhang and colleagues[33] reviewed 256 patients with supracondylar humerus fractures treated with closed or open reduction and Kirschner wire fixation and found a 14.8% loss of reduction. They identified poor surgical technique as the largest risk factor for loss of reduction but also identified BMI greater than 25 kg/m^2, lateral-only pin constructs, and Gartland type 3 fractures as significantly increasing the risk for loss of reduction. Chang and colleagues[34] performed a similar study of 107 children with type 3 supracondylar humerus fractures and found that obese children were more likely to develop postoperative loss of reduction and varus alignment.

These studies highlight the potential pitfalls of caring for obese children with fractures of the distal humerus. Obese children have been consistently shown to have a higher rate of preoperative and postoperative complications in

the treatment of supracondylar humerus fractures. Understanding the increased risk of displacement may lower a surgeon's threshold for an open reduction to achieve a more perfect reduction or the placement of a medial pin. These considerations must be weighed against the potential increased difficulty of finding surface anatomic landmarks and visualizing during exposure in the obese patient with a swollen elbow.

LOWER EXTREMITY

Lower extremity fractures have also been shown to have an increased incidence and severity in the obese pediatric population. In 2008, Pollack and colleagues[35] published a review of survey data from the parents of 3232 children involved in 2873 motor vehicle collisions. Their analysis identified increased odds of sustaining an injury to the extremities within the overweight and obese populations (OR 2.64; 95% CI, 1.64–4.77 and OR 2.54; 95% CI, 1.15–5.59, respectively). Further analysis of their data seemed to suggest that obese children tended to sustain fractures in the distal portions of long bones while the normal and underweight populations tended to fracture the femur, pelvis, and clavicle. This finding of an increased risk of distal fractures was replicated by Gilbert and colleagues,[24] when they reviewed the trauma registries for 2 trauma centers for pediatric lower extremity long bone fractures. They identified 331 patients with a total of 397 long bone fractures and found that obese patients were twice as likely (relative risk [RR] 2.20; 95% CI, 1.25–3.89) to have fractures involving the physis. The etiology is unclear but could be related to mechanical or hormonal effects. Kessler and colleagues[21] performed a population-based cohort study of 913,178 patients ages 2 years to 19 years. All patients were categorized into 5 weight cohorts and their charts reviewed for lower extremity fractures. In total, 7158 lower extremity fractures were identified and a clear linear relationship was found between patient weight and risk for fracture. This relationship persisted across genders and all examined age groups. They found that the extremely obese ($\geq$1.2 × 95th percentile for age BMI or BMI >35 kg/m^2) had a 1.4 odds of fracture whereas the moderately obese (>95th percentile for age BMI and <1.2 × 95th percentile BMI or BMI 30–35 kg/m^2) had a 1.23 odds of sustaining a fracture compared with normal-weight individuals.

Leet and colleagues[36] first noted an increased rate of complications when caring for obese children with femur fractures in 2005. Over the following years, several studies were published showing an increased risk of loss of reduction when treating femur fractures in children weighing more than 48 kg to 50 kg with titanium elastic nails.[37,38] This has been recently challenged by Shaha and colleagues[39] when they demonstrated no difference in radiographic angulation or union when treating children with stainless steel flexible intramedullary nails. Despite these findings, locked reamed intramedullary nail fixation is a biomechanically better choice if the bone size and skeletal maturity permit. Although obesity is frequently cited as a reason for caution when treating pediatric femur fractures with spica casting,[40,41] only 1 study has compared obese and nonobese patients and found no difference in skin complications.[42]

Technical tips

- Consider use of stronger stainless steel flexible nails or locked intramedullary nails for femur fractures in obese patients.
- Obesity does not seem to be a contraindication for spica cast treatment of femur fractures.

Tibia fractures have not demonstrated a similar weight limitation for titanium elastic nails. Goodbody and colleagues[43] reviewed a cohort of 95 adolescents with tibia fractures and did not find a significant difference in the rate of malunion or time to healing between those over 50 kg and those under 50 kg. Additionally, Fedorack and colleagues[44] examined the effect of BMI on complications relating to external fixation of lower extremities for a variety of conditions (deformity, lengthening, and trauma), and found that obesity did not alter the rate of complication when all cases were considered. They did not evaluate fracture treatment separately. Consideration should also be given to another potential complication of external fixation—weight gain during treatment—which averaged 0.25 kg/wk.[45] The authors frequently

counsel patients regarding this likelihood and the need to decrease caloric intake while energy expenditures are decreased due to immobility.

Although fractures of the foot and ankle were found to have the strongest correlation with obesity in Kessler and colleagues' population study,[21] little has been published about the treatment of specific injury patterns or modifications of treatment due to obesity. Nevertheless, it seems intuitive that obese patients likely require additional assistance to mobilize due to increased weight and lower relative strength, balance, and coordination.[46] Additionally, the additional force of weight bearing with excess weight may necessitate a higher level of immobilization for patient tolerance or more delayed weight bearing to prevent fracture displacement.

Tips: surgical considerations for lower extremity fracture cases

Additional discussion of some general surgical principles in lower extremity obesity surgery is warranted. First, ensure an appropriate operating table is available. Some older fracture tops are rated for only 136 kg. These may flex excessively during fracture surgery, especially when using impact devices or applying forceful traction or compression. Many newer tops are now reinforced and rated for 227 kg. Although not specifically recommended, if there is excessive flexing of a radiolucent top, applying an adjustable stool underneath the top may provide additional support.

Another challenge may be tourniquet application on large, conical thighs. One maneuver described is to pull traction on the fat and apply the tourniquet proximal, thereby displacing the proximal thigh roll distal to the edge of the tourniquet.[47] An additional maneuver that the authors have used is to apply adhesive circumferentially to the thigh and then apply longitudinal strips of tape to the area underneath the tourniquet, leaving quite a bit of length. The padding and tourniquet are then applied and the tape is then reflected back over the tourniquet and secured to the thigh or pannus above (Fig. 1). The origin of this method could not be determined and no reference for its application could be found.

SPINE INJURIES

Several studies of trauma registries, including those by Rana and colleagues[3] and Witt and

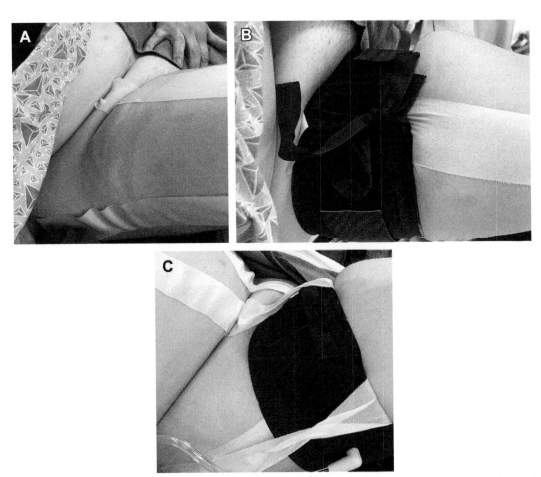

Fig. 1. An alternative tourniquet application technique for obese thighs. (*A*) Apply benzoin to the thigh, followed by vertical tape strips. (*B*) Apply tourniquet over the tape strips while pulling the fat distally. (*C*) Reflect the tape back up over the tourniquet and secure to thigh or pannus proximal to tourniquet.

colleagues,[1] have noted that obesity seems protective against injuries to the spine, solid organs, and head. Aside from these broad generalizations, there is a dearth of evidence suggesting any unique pattern of spinal trauma in obese pediatric patients. With regard to treatment, no specific studies have been published but some inferences can be made. If bracing is required, there may be concerns regarding brace tolerance and efficacy. Data from scoliosis bracing suggest that obesity is associated with poor curve correction and poor brace compliance[48,49] These difficulties are likely due to the increased distance to and tissue interposed between the skin and the bony structures targeted for force application. In the management of spine fractures, the corrective force applied may not be as critical as preventing additional overloading, and so success might be expected if an appropriately

fitting brace is able to be applied and compliance is achieved.

Similarly, there are no data on spine fracture surgical outcomes and obesity. Positioning challenges may be encountered, and a Jackson spine table with a variety of hip and chest pads may be helpful. In addition, an adjustable head holder is helpful for achieving neutral cervical spine alignment and avoiding ocular pressure, because obesity has been shown to be a risk factor for vision loss.[50] Data from scoliosis surgeries suggest increased rates of infection may be expected.[51,52]

Technical tips: spine surgery

- Pay close attention to positioning.
- Consider additional maneuvers for infection prevention: higher antibiotic dosing and local antibiotics.

SUMMARY

Obese children and adolescents who sustain high-energy injuries may present with more severe injuries, more extremity injuries, and higher ISSs. They are at increased risk for complications, prolonged ventilation, and ICU stay and have increased mortality. Inflammatory response to polytrauma may be exaggerated in obese patients. Childhood obesity is associated with altered bone structure and bone mass accrual, and obese patients have higher fracture rates and are more likely to sustain growth plate fractures in the lower extremity compared with nonobese children. Obese patients have a higher risk of loss of reduction of forearm fractures. At the elbow, obesity is associated with more severe supracondylar fractures and a higher likelihood of lateral condyle fractures. In the lower extremities, obese patients are more likely to have complications with femur fractures and have higher rates of foot and ankle fracture. Particular attention is needed to cast application and monitoring of fracture alignment for nonoperative treatment. For surgical treatment, special consideration may be needed for positioning, implant choice, and infection prevention.

REFERENCES

1. Witt CE, Arbabi S, Nathens AB, et al. Obesity in pediatric trauma. J Pediatr Surg 2017;52(4):628–32.
2. Alselaim N, Malaekah H, Saade M, et al. Does obesity impact the pattern and outcome of trauma in children? J Pediatr Surg 2012;47(7):1404–9.
3. Rana AR, Michalsky MP, Teich S, et al. Childhood obesity: a risk factor for injuries observed at a level-1 trauma center. J Pediatr Surg 2009;44(8):1601–5.
4. Brown CV, Neville AL, Salim A, et al. The impact of obesity on severely injured children and adolescents. J Pediatr Surg 2006;41(1):88–91 [discussion: 88–91].
5. Backstrom IC, MacLennan PA, Sawyer JR, et al. Pediatric obesity and traumatic lower-extremity long-bone fracture outcomes. J Trauma Acute Care Surg 2012;73(4):966–71.
6. Vaughan N, Tweed J, Greenwell C, et al. The impact of morbid obesity on solid organ injury in children using the ATOMAC protocol at a pediatric level I trauma center. J Pediatr Surg 2017;52(2):345–8.
7. Kim JE, Hsieh MH, Shum PC, et al. Risk and injury severity of obese child passengers in motor vehicle crashes. Obesity (Silver Spring) 2015;23(3):644–52.
8. Goh VL, Wakeham MK, Brazauskas R, et al. Obesity is not associated with increased mortality and morbidity in critically ill children. JPEN J Parenter Enteral Nutr 2013;37(1):102–8.
9. Ross E, Burris A, Murphy JT. Obesity and outcomes following burns in the pediatric population. J Pediatr Surg 2014;49(3):469–73.
10. Romano T, Koutroulis I, Weiner E, et al. Comparison of resource utilization and length of hospitalization between overweight and healthy-weight pediatric trauma patients presenting to a pediatric emergency department with moderate to severe injury: a prospective study. Pediatr Emerg Care 2017. [Epub ahead of print].
11. Fleming-Dutra KE, Mao J, Leonard JC. Acute care costs in overweight children: a pediatric urban cohort study. Child Obes 2013;9(4):338–45.
12. Cole ZA, Harvey NC, Kim M, et al, Southampton Women's Survey Study Group. Increased fat mass is associated with increased bone size but reduced volumetric density in pre pubertal children. Bone 2012;50:562–7.
13. Vandewalle S, Taes Y, Van Helvoirt M, et al. Bone size and bone strength are increased in obese male adolescents. J Clin Endocrinol Metab 2013;98(7):3019–28.
14. Júnior IF, Cardoso JR, Christofaro DG, et al. The relationship between visceral fat thickness and bone mineral density in sedentary obese children and adolescents. BMC Pediatr 2013;13:37.
15. Wey HE, Binkley TL, Beare TM, et al. Cross-sectional versus longitudinal associations of lean and fat mass with pQCT bone outcomes in children. J Clin Endocrinol Metab 2011;96(1):106–14.
16. Dimitri P, Bishop N, Walsh JS, et al. Obesity is a risk factor for fracture in children but is protective against fracture in adults: a paradox. Bone 2012;50:457–66.
17. Golden NH, Abrams SA, Committee on Nutrition. Optimizing bone health in children and adolescents. Pediatrics 2014;134(4):e1229–43.
18. Valerio G, Gallè F, Mancusi C, et al. Prevalence of overweight in children with bone fractures: a case control study. BMC Pediatr 2012;12:166.
19. Manning Ryan L, Teach SJ, Searcy K, et al. The association between weight status and pediatric forearm fractures resulting from ground-level falls. Pediatr Emerg Care 2015;31(12):835–8.
20. Adams AL, Kessler JI, Deramerian K, et al. Associations between childhood obesity and upper and lower extremity injuries. Inj Prev 2013;19(3):191–7.
21. Kessler J, Koebnick C, Smith N, et al. Childhood obesity is associated with increased risk of most lower extremity fractures. Clin Orthop Relat Res 2013;471(4):1199–207.
22. Turner RW, Perrin EM, Coyne-Beasley T, et al. Reported sports participation, race, sex, ethnicity, and obesity in US adolescents from NHANES physical activity (PAQ_D). Glob Pediatr Health 2015;2. 2333794X15577944.

23. Kwan C, Doan Q, Oliveria JP, et al. Do obese children experience more severe fractures than nonobese children? A cross-sectional study from a paediatric emergency department. Paediatr Child Health 2014;19(5):251–5.

24. Gilbert SR, MacLennan PA, Backstrom I, et al. Altered lower extremity fracture characteristics in obese pediatric trauma patients. J Orthop Trauma 2015;29(1):e12–7.

25. Pomerantz WJ, Timm NL, Gittelman MA. Injury patterns in obese versus nonobese children presenting to a pediatric emergency department. Pediatrics 2010;125(4):681–5.

26. Ryan LM, Teach SJ, Ezeibe U, et al. Is high weight status associated with pediatric forearm fractures requiring anatomic reduction? J Investig Med 2015;63(4):649–52.

27. Hirsch DG, Tyo J, Wrotniak BH. Desaturation in procedural sedation for children with long bone fractures: does weight status matter? Am J Emerg Med 2017;35(8):1060–3.

28. Auer RT, Mazzone P, Robinson L, et al. Childhood obesity increases the risk of failure in the treatment of distal forearm fractures. J Pediatr Orthop 2016; 36(8):e86–8.

29. DeFrancesco CJ, Rogers BH, Shah AS. Obesity increases risk of loss of reduction after casting for diaphyseal fractures of the radius and ulna in children: an observational cohort study. J Orthop Trauma 2018;32:e46–51.

30. Okoroafor UC, Cannada LK, McGinty JL. Obesity and failure of nonsurgical management of pediatric both-bone forearm fractures. J Hand Surg Am 2017;42(9):711–6.

31. Fornari ED, Suszter M, Roocroft J, et al. Childhood obesity as a risk factor for lateral condyle fractures over supracondylar humerus fractures. Clin Orthop Relat Res 2013;471(4):1193–8.

32. Seeley MA, Gagnier JJ, Srinivasan RC, et al. Obesity and its effects on pediatric supracondylar humeral fractures. J Bone Joint Surg Am 2014; 96(3):e18.

33. Sangkomkamhang T, Singjam U, Leeprakobboon D. Risk factors for loss of fixation in pediatric supracondylar humeral fractures. J Med Assoc Thai 2014; 97(Suppl 9):S23–8.

34. Chang CH, Kao HK, Lee WC, et al. Influence of obesity on surgical outcomes in type III paediatric supracondylar humeral fractures. Injury 2015;46(11):2181–4.

35. Pollack KM, Xie D, Arbogast KB, et al. Body mass index and injury risk among US children 9-15 years old in motor vehicle crashes. Inj Prev 2008;14(6):366–71.

36. Leet AI, Pichard CP, Ain MC. Surgical treatment of femoral fractures in obese children: does excessive body weight increase the rate of complications? J Bone Joint Surg Am 2005;87(12):2609–13.

37. Li Y, Stabile KJ, Shilt JS. Biomechanical analysis of titanium elastic nail fixation in a pediatric femur fracture model. J Pediatr Orthop 2008;28(8):874–8.

38. Weiss JM, Choi P, Ghatan C, et al. Complications with flexible nailing of femur fractures more than double with child obesity and weight >50 kg. J Child Orthop 2009;3(1):53–8.

39. Shaha J, Cage JM, Black S, et al. Flexible intramedullary nails for femur fractures in pediatric patients heavier than 100 pounds. J Pediatr Orthop 2018;38:88–93.

40. Czertak DJ, Hennrikus WL. The treatment of pediatric femur fractures with early 90-90 spica casting. J Pediatr Orthop 1999;19(2):229–32.

41. Henderson OL, Morrissy RT, Gerdes MH, et al. Early casting of femoral shaft fractures in children. J Pediatr Orthop 1984;4(1):16–21.

42. DiFazio R, Vessey J, Zurakowski D, et al. Incidence of skin complications and associated charges in children treated with hip spica casts for femur fractures. J Pediatr Orthop 2011;31(1):17–22.

43. Goodbody CM, Lee RJ, Flynn JM, et al. Titanium elastic nailing for pediatric tibia fractures: do older, heavier kids do worse? J Pediatr Orthop 2016;36(5):472–7.

44. Fedorak GT, Cuomo AV, Otsuka NY. Does pediatric body mass index affect surgical outcomes of lower-extremity external fixation? J Pediatr Orthop 2015;35(4):391–4.

45. Culotta BA, Gilbert SR, Sawyer JR, et al. Weight gain during external fixation. J Child Orthop 2013;7(2):147–50.

46. Goulding A, Jones IE, Taylor RW, et al. Dynamic and static tests of balance and postural sway in boys: effects of previous wrist bone fractures and high adiposity. Gait Posture 2003;17(2):136–41.

47. Krackow KA. A maneuver for improved positioning of a tourniquet in the obese patient. Clin Orthop Relat Res 1982;(168):80–2.

48. Goodbody CM, Asztalos IB, Sankar WN, et al. It's not just the big kids: both high and low BMI impact bracing success for adolescent idiopathic scoliosis. J Child Orthop 2016;10(5):395–404.

49. Zaina F, Donzelli S, Negrini S. Overweight is not predictive of bracing failure in adolescent idiopathic scoliosis: results from a retrospective cohort study. Eur Spine J 2017;26(6):1670–5.

50. Su AW, Lin SC, Larson AN. Perioperative vision loss in spine surgery and other orthopaedic procedures. J Am Acad Orthop Surg 2016;24(10):702–10.

51. Katyal C, Grossman S, Dworkin A, et al. Increased risk of infection in obese adolescents after pedicle screw instrumentation for idiopathic scoliosis. Spine Deform 2015;3(2):166–71.

52. De la Garza Ramos R, Nakhla J, Nasser R, et al. Effect of body mass index on surgical outcomes after posterior spinal fusion for adolescent idiopathic scoliosis. Neurosurg Focus 2017;43(4):E5.

Hand and Wrist

The Impact of Obesity on Orthopedic Upper Extremity Surgery

Jon Cooper Wall Jr, MD[a], Hillary Powers Wall, BS[b],
Bradley O. Osemwengie, BS[b],
Brendan J. MacKay, MD[a,c,*]

KEYWORDS

- Obesity • Hand • Upper extremity • Surgery • Complication • Management
- Carpal tunnel syndrome • Arthritis

KEY POINTS

- Obesity is widespread in America and has effects on all medical specialties, including surgery of the hand and upper extremity.
- Obese patients are at risk for injuries of the upper extremity, carpal tunnel syndrome, and hand and wrist osteoarthritis.
- Intraoperative and anesthetic considerations should include the physiology of the obese as well as patient positioning and regional anesthetic difficulties, and perioperative antibiotics should be considered.
- Postoperative complications can include fracture healing complications, including malunion, and wound healing issues, including infection.
- Some recent literature suggests surgery of the hand and upper extremity may be somewhat immune to the postoperative complications seen in other regions of the body.
- There is limited literature that evaluates the postoperative complications and outcomes specific to hand and upper extremity surgery.

INTRODUCTION

The prevalence of obesity is increasing in the United States[1] (Figs. 1 and 2). It is estimated that approximately one-third (36.5%) of adult Americans are obese, defined as body mass index (BMI) greater than 30 kg/m². The obesity rate is higher among middle aged (40–59 years) and older adults (>60 years) than among younger adults (20–39 years).[2] The prevalence of obesity differs with race, sex, and socioeconomic status. Women of higher socioeconomic status are less likely to be obese, whereas non-Hispanic black and Mexican-American men of higher socioeconomic status are likely to have obesity.[3] No statistically significant correlations have been identified between level of education and obesity in men. However, there is a significant correlation among women, showing that women with a college education are less likely to have obesity compared with women who are less educated.[4] Patients with higher BMIs have a greater likelihood of experiencing comorbid health conditions.[4,5] These comorbidities can negatively affect the

Disclosure: None of the authors have any relationships with a commercial company that has a direct financial interest in the subject matter or materials discussed in the article or with a company making a competing product.
[a] Department of Orthopaedic Surgery, Texas Tech University Health Sciences Center, Mail Stop 9436, 3601 4th Street, Lubbock, TX 79430, USA; [b] Office of Student Affairs, Texas Tech University Health Sciences Center School of Medicine, Mail Stop 6222, 3601 4th Street, Lubbock, TX 79430, USA; [c] UMC Health System, 602 Indiana Avenue, Lubbock, TX 79415, USA
* Corresponding author. Orthopaedic Hand Clinic, Medical Office Plaza (MOP) II, 808 Joliet, Suite 210, Lubbock, TX 79415, USA.
E-mail address: brendan.j.mackay@ttuhsc.edu

Orthop Clin N Am 49 (2018) 345–351
https://doi.org/10.1016/j.ocl.2018.02.008
0030-5898/18/© 2018 Elsevier Inc. All rights reserved.

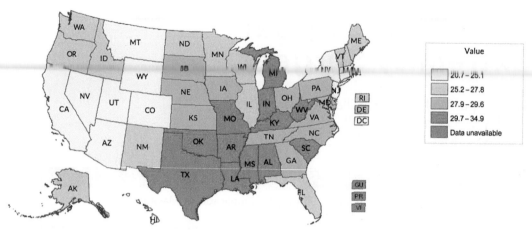

Fig. 1. Percentage of adults with obesity in 2011. Obese is defined as a body mass index (BMI) greater than or equal to 30; BMI was calculated from self-report weight and height (kg/m^2). Respondents reporting weight less than 23 kg (50 pounds) or greater than or equal to 295 kg (650 pounds), height less than 90 cm (3 feet) or greater than or equal to 240 cm (8 feet), or BMI less than 12 and greater than or equal to 100 were excluded. (*From* Centers for Disease Control and Prevention (CDC). National Center for Chronic Disease Prevention and Health Promotion, Division of Nutrition, Physical Activity, and Obesity. Data, trends and maps [online]. Available at: https://www.cdc.gov/nccdphp/dnpao/data-trends-maps/index.html. Accessed January 01, 2018.)

health of obese patients and increase the cost of care compared with the nonobese population.[2] Given the prevalence of obesity and the continued societal pressure to provide high-quality care at low cost, physicians need to familiarize themselves with considerations pertinent to their specialty for proper management and treatment of obese patients.[6] Research across a myriad of medical specialties is available to guide treatment.[7] The orthopedic literature has shown that implementation of specific perioperative measures makes it possible for virtually all obese patients to undergo indicated orthopedic procedures.[8] These measures can reduce difficulties often encountered while performing procedures on obese patients, leading to better outcomes, pain relief, and better quality of life for patients.[9] This article specifically reviews the existing literature on obesity and its impact on orthopedic upper extremity surgery.

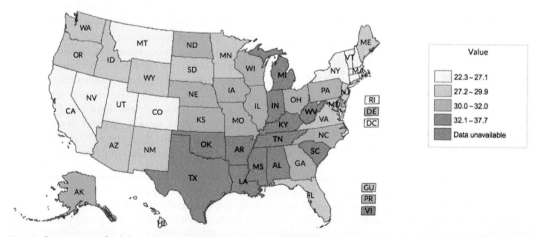

Fig. 2. Percentage of adults with obesity in 2016. Obese is defined as a BMI greater than or equal to 30; BMI was calculated from self-report weight and height (kg/m^2). Respondents reporting weight less than 23 kg (50 pounds) or greater than or equal to 295 kg (650 pounds), height less than 90 cm (3 feet) or greater than or equal to 240 cm (8 feet), or BMI less than 12 and greater than or equal to 100 were excluded (*From* Centers for Disease Control and Prevention (CDC). National Center for Chronic Disease Prevention and Health Promotion, Division of Nutrition, Physical Activity, and Obesity. Data, trends and maps [online]. Available at: https://www.cdc.gov/nccdphp/dnpao/data-trends-maps/index.html. Accessed January 01, 2018.)

DISCUSSION

Medical Considerations

Obesity is a risk factor for venous thromboembolism (VTE), diabetes mellitus, hypertension (HTN), cardiovascular disease, pulmonary disease, obstructive sleep apnea, metabolic syndrome, and even some psychiatric ailments.[2,10,11] All of these conditions can significantly magnify the risks of nonsurgical and surgical treatments and complicate the perioperative period, even if the patient is receiving appropriate medical treatment of their health issues. It is imperative that a complete, accurate medical history including current medications and a list of previous adverse events is obtained for each patient. Patients should be questioned on their compliance with necessary, regularly scheduled primary care and specialist visits and screening laboratory work. If surgery is being considered, patients should have a preanesthesia evaluation to determine whether any medical optimization is needed.

Orthopedic Considerations

Obese patients are at increased risk for degenerative joint disease.[12] This risk was initially documented in weight-bearing joints (hip and knee) and was thought to be the result of increased joint forces[12] Since that time, an increased incidence of degenerative joint changes has been documented in non–weight-bearing joints (hand and wrist) of obese patients.[13] As a result, systemic metabolic pathophysiology is being recognized as the culprit rather than strictly mechanical causes.[14]

It has also been documented in the literature that there is an increase in the incidence of carpal tunnel syndrome in the obese population,[15–17] with one meta-analysis showing overweight patients to have an increased risk of carpal tunnel release 1.5-fold and obese patients 2-fold.[18] Although diabetes mellitus was thought to be the reason for the increased risk of carpal tunnel syndrome, it was found not to be an independent risk factor when adjusted for BMI.[19] Although the severity of nerve conduction studies increased as age increased, it did not increase as severity of BMI increased.[20] Despite this correlation with BMI, patients who undergo significant weight loss did not have significant improvement in nerve conduction studies.[21]

Obese patients may be at higher risk of sustaining orthopedic trauma. One study found that a BMI of 25 to 30 increases a patient's odds of sustaining an orthopedic injury by 15%, whereas a BMI of 40 or greater increases a patient's odds of an orthopedic injury by 48%.[22] Another study found that obese women

have a higher incidence of humerus fractures than those of normal BMI.[23] This increased risk has been attributed to mechanical and physiologic factors. Obese patients are at higher risk of falling and are also less able to protect against fall.[24–26] When they fall, they are more likely to fall backward or sideways instead of forward, which decreases their ability to control their fall[25,27] (**Table 1**). Weight loss has been shown to be associated with an increase in fracture risk of the previously obese.[28–31] This increased risk may be explained by the loss of bone stock previously stimulated by the routine bearing of additional weight. It is thought that this may be attenuated with an exercise program to correspond with calorie restriction. Adiponectin, one of the cytokines produced by adipocytes, is known to have a deleterious effect on bone. Its levels have been shown to be higher in overweight women with a fracture than in those without a fracture[32] and it may be a future target for predicting fracture risk in obese patients.[23] Furthermore, obese patients tend to have lower 25-hydroxyvitamin D levels and may need higher doses of supplementation to achieve adequate serum levels.[33] Low levels may decrease bone density and increase fracture risk.

Table 1	
Risk factors associated with fractures in obese patients	
Risk Factor	
Reported in Women	**Reported in Men**
Age	Previous fracture
Previous fracture	Mobility limitations
Maternal hip fracture	Difficulty climbing
Low bone mineral	10 steps
density[a]	Difficulty walking
Use of arms to assist	2 blocks
stand from a	Narrow walk pace
sitting position	
Falls	
Two or more in	
the previous year	
Poor or fair general	
health	
Glucocorticoid use	
Comorbidities	
Asthma	
Emphysema	
Diabetes with	
insulin use	

[a] Odds ratio 1.6 (95% confidence interval 1.5,1.8) per 1 standard deviation decrease at femoral neck.

From Premaor MO, Comim FV, Compston JE. Obesity and fractures. Arq Bras Endocrinol Metab 2014;58(5):472; with permission.

Intraoperative/Anesthetic Considerations

Some obese patients either exceed the 230-kg (500-pound) weight limit of a standard operating room table are too large in width to be stable on a single bed. In this instance, if available, a specialized operating room table that can bear up to 460 kg (1000 pounds) may be used. Otherwise, 2 standard tables can be placed side by side with adequate results.[34]

Special attention needs to be paid to preoperative positioning. If possible, patients should be allowed to position themselves on the operating table, receiving help only as needed.[8] Positions that restrict abdominal and chest wall expansion should be avoided because they may compromise ventilation in obese patients.[35] Improper positioning can also lead to peripheral nerve injuries. Excessive abduction, extension, or rotation of the upper extremity as well as poor positioning of the arm boards can cause injuries to the brachial plexus.[34] Many of these problems can be mitigated with the help of multiple staff personnel as well as appropriate size of equipment for the individual. Generous padding on the equipment should also be used in order to reduce the amount of pressure placed on certain parts of the body.[36]

Anesthesia management of obese patients is affected by both physiologic and anatomic challenges. Anatomic features may be altered from excess adipose tissue hindering palpation of osseous landmarks, creating difficulties that range from simple intravenous access to regional blocks.[8] This consideration in hand and upper extremity surgery is important because many procedures are done under regional anesthesia. Anesthesia providers need experience with longer needles[37] and have to consider dosing requirements based on ideal and actual body weights, including perioperative antibiotics.[38–41] This view is supported by a study of more than 2000 supraclavicular blocks that showed residents had a significantly less successful rate of block (80% in nonobese, 73% in obese), whereas there was only a slight decrease in the overall success rate of more experienced providers (97.3% in nonobese, 94.3% in obese). This finding shows that although obesity does make the regional block more difficult, it is still worth pursuing.[42]

Postoperative Considerations

Obesity is also an independent risk factor for VTE and pulmonary embolism (PE).[43–46] Although hand and upper extremity procedures are shorter procedures, more likely to undergo regional anesthesia, and generally allow immediate postoperative ambulation, the risk of a thromboembolic event is still present and mechanical VTE prophylaxis is recommended at minimum.[43] It is also interesting to note that, despite the lower extremity being a more common site for VTE overall, obese patients are also at risk for deep vein thrombosis (DVT) of the upper extremity.[47] However, this is still not a common occurrence, and although there are no formal recommendations, risk of VTE in a patient undergoing upper extremity surgery likely does not need chemical VTE prophylaxis. The surgeon should evaluate the patient's clinical picture and stratify the patient by risk to determine whether chemical VTE prophylaxis should be used in conjunction with mechanical VTE prophylaxis.

Surgical Complications and Outcomes

There is extensive literature showing a relationship between obesity and postoperative complications, especially in orthopedics.[48–51] These complications include such things as surgical site infections, prosthetic and hardware failure, fracture malunion, DVT, PEs, and postoperative hypoxemia.[8,52] This association has often been extrapolated to hand and upper extremity surgery, but it has only recently been studied in isolation. A recent case-control study investigated measures of postoperative complications, including infection, wound problems, nerve dysfunction, and reoperation, and found that there was no significant association between obese and nonobese patients and postoperative complications (Table 2). These results, compared with other areas of the body, are unique in their lack of significant association with obesity and postoperative complications, which may be caused by many factors, including that hand surgeries are usually done under regional rather than general anesthesia, do not significantly impair the mobility of the patient, and there is proportionately less subcutaneous tissue in the upper extremity as opposed to the lower extremity, reducing the chance of hematoma formation. Whatever the reason, this is contrary to what has previously been assumed from extrapolated data and shows that further research should be conducted to better understand this relationship as it relates specifically to the upper extremity.

When considering all fractures, the literature shows an increase in morbidity and complications in the obese population, including nonunion, longer recovery, and a higher prevalence of comorbidities.[48,53–56] Even when adjusted for age, comorbidities, and high-impact fractures, these patients were found to have longer

Table 2
Procedure categories and the number and description of complications that occurred in both the obese and nonobese groups

Procedure Category	Complications in the Obese Croup; N (%)	Complications in the Nonobese Group; N (%)	P Value[a]
Bony	17 (15) Antibiotics for infection: 9 Delayed incision healing: 2 Nerve injury: 2 Wound dehiscence: 2 Hematoma: 2 Reoperation: 6	18 (15) Antibiotics for infection: 6 Delayed incision healing: 1 Nerve injury: 2 Wound dehiscence: 0 Hematoma: 1 Reoperation: 12	.92
Nerve	10 (6) Antibiotics for infection: 6 Delayed incision healing: 3 Nerve injury: 0 Wound dehiscence: 3 Hematoma: 2 Reoperation: 1	7 (4) Antibiotics for infection: 4 Delayed incision healing: 1 Nerve injury: 0 Wound dehiscence: 2 Hematoma: 1 Reoperation: 1	.38
Soft tissue	9 (6) Antibiotics for infection: 8 Delayed incision healing: 5 Nerve injury: 3 Wound dehiscence: 2 Hematoma: 2 Reoperation: 1	14 (10) Antibiotics for infection: 6 Delayed incision healing: 3 Nerve injury: 0 Wound dehiscence: 2 Hematoma: 1 Reoperation: 6	.29

Total numbers (%) for each procedure category is number of patients. Individual patients may have experienced multiple types of complications.
[a] P from χ^2 analyses.
From London DA, Stepan JG, Lalchandani GR, et al. The impact of obesity on complications of elbow, forearm, and hand surgeries. J Hand Surg Am 2014;39(8):1582; with permission.

hospital stays than their nonobese counterparts[57] as well as worse quality-of-life questionnaire scores both before and after fracture.[57]

With regard to the upper extremity, obesity was shown to be associated with increased postoperative complications in the operative management of humeral shaft fractures, including both local (stiffness, infection) and systemic (DVT, PE, acute myocardial infarction, respiratory failure, acute renal failure) complications as well as mortality at 6 months, 1 year, and 2 years after surgery.[58]

SUMMARY

Comprehensive review of the literature confirms that obesity is an important risk factor to consider in orthopedic care. Although literature continues to evolve and grow, there is a paucity of studies focused on orthopedic upper extremity care. At the moment, clinicians are forced to extrapolate data from other parts of the body to supplement the literature on obesity and upper extremity orthopedic care. However, there are some suggestions in the current literature that

the upper limb distal to the shoulder may be immune to some of the complications and worse outcomes seen in other areas. This possibility will need to be the focus of future research.

REFERENCES

1. Behavioral Risk Factor Surveillance System. Nutrition, physical activity, and obesity: data, trends and maps. 2017. Available at: https://www.cdc.gov/nccdphp/dnpao/data-trends-maps/index.html. Accessed January 1, 2017.
2. US Centers for Disease Control and Prevention. Adult obesity facts. 2017. Available at: https://www.cdc.gov/obesity/data/adult.html. Accessed December 7, 2017.
3. Ogden CL, Lamb MM, Carrol MD, et al. Obesity and socioeconomic status in adults: United States 1988-1994 and 2005-2008. Hyattsville (MD): National Center for Health Statistics; 2010.
4. Ogden CL, Lamb MM, Carroll MD, et al. Obesity and socioeconomic status in adults: United States, 2005-2008. NCHS Data Brief 2010;(50):1–8.
5. Ogden CL, Lamb MM, Carroll MD, et al. Obesity and socioeconomic status in children and adolescents:

United States, 2005-2008. NCHS Data Brief 2010;(51): 1–8.

6. Grace D. Surgery for obesity. 2nd edition. New York: Oxford University Press; 2000.

7. Youdim A. The clinician's guide to the treatment of obesity. New York: Springer; 2015.

8. Guss D, Bhattacharyya T. Perioperative management of the obese orthopaedic patient. J Am Acad Orthop Surg 2006;14(7):425–32.

9. Mihalko WM, Bergin PF, Kelly FB, et al. Obesity, orthopaedics, and outcomes. J Am Acad Orthop Surg 2014;22(11):683–90.

10. Li Z, Bowerman S, Heber D. Health ramifications of the obesity epidemic. Surg Clin North Am 2005; 85(4):681–701, v.

11. Berrington de Gonzalez A, Hartge P, Cerhan JR, et al. Body-mass index and mortality among 1.46 million white adults. N Engl J Med 2010;363(23): 2211–9.

12. Bourne R, Mukhi S, Zhu N, et al. Role of obesity on the risk for total hip or knee arthroplasty. Clin Orthop Relat Res 2007;465:185–8.

13. Yusuf E, Nelissen RG, Ioan-Facsinay A, et al. Association between weight or body mass index and hand osteoarthritis: a systematic review. Ann Rheum Dis 2010;69(4):761–5.

14. Sellam J, Berenbaum F. Is osteoarthritis a metabolic disease? Joint Bone Spine 2013;80(6):568–73.

15. Kouyoumdjian JA, Morita MD, Rocha PR, et al. Body mass index and carpal tunnel syndrome. Arq Neuropsiquiatr 2000;58(2A):252–6.

16. Geoghegan JM, Clark DI, Bainbridge LC, et al. Risk factors in carpal tunnel syndrome. J Hand Surg Br 2004;29(4):315–20.

17. Stallings SP, Kasdan ML, Soergel TM, et al. A case-control study of obesity as a risk factor for carpal tunnel syndrome in a population of 600 patients presenting for independent medical examination. J Hand Surg Am 1997;22(2):211–5.

18. Shiri R, Pourmemari MH, Falah-Hassani K, et al. The effect of excess body mass on the risk of carpal tunnel syndrome: a meta-analysis of 58 studies. Obes Rev 2015;16(12):1094–104.

19. Becker J, Nora DB, Gomes I, et al. An evaluation of gender, obesity, age and diabetes mellitus as risk factors for carpal tunnel syndrome. Clin Neurophysiol 2002;113(9):1429–34.

20. Kouyoumdjian JA, Zanetta DM, Morita MP. Evaluation of age, body mass index, and wrist index as risk factors for carpal tunnel syndrome severity. Muscle Nerve 2002;25(1):93–7.

21. Kurt S, Kisacik B, Kaplan Y, et al. Obesity and carpal tunnel syndrome: is there a causal relationship? Eur Neurol 2008;59(5):253–7.

22. Finkelstein EA, Chen H, Prabhu M, et al. The relationship between obesity and injuries among U.S. adults. Am J Health Promot 2007;21(5):460–8.

23. Premaor MO, Comim FV, Compston JE. Obesity and fractures. Arq Bras Endocrinol Metabol 2014; 58(5):470–7.

24. Chan BK, Marshall LM, Winters KM, et al. Incident fall risk and physical activity and physical performance among older men: the Osteoporotic Fractures in Men study. Am J Epidemiol 2007;165(6): 696–703.

25. Corbeil P, Simoneau M, Rancourt D, et al. Increased risk for falling associated with obesity: mathematical modeling of postural control. IEEE Trans Neural Syst Rehabil Eng 2001;9(2):126–36.

26. Ensrud KE, Ewing SK, Taylor BC, et al. Comparison of 2 frailty indexes for prediction of falls, disability, fractures, and death in older women. Arch Intern Med 2008;168(4):382–9.

27. Mignardot JB, Olivier I, Promayon E, et al. Obesity impact on the attentional cost for controlling posture. PLoS One 2010;5(12):e14387.

28. Cummings SR, Nevitt MC. Non-skeletal determinants of fractures: the potential importance of the mechanics of falls. Study of Osteoporotic Fractures Research Group. Osteoporos Int 1994;4(Suppl 1): 67–70.

29. Langlois JA, Harris T, Looker AC, et al. Weight change between age 50 years and old age is associated with risk of hip fracture in white women aged 67 years and older. Arch Intern Med 1996;156(9): 989–94.

30. Meyer HE, Tverdal A, Selmer R. Weight variability, weight change and the incidence of hip fracture: a prospective study of 39,000 middle-aged Norwegians. Osteoporos Int 1998;8(4):373–8.

31. Ensrud KE, Ewing SK, Stone KL, et al. Intentional and unintentional weight loss increase bone loss and hip fracture risk in older women. J Am Geriatr Soc 2003;51(12):1740–7.

32. Barbour KE, Zmuda JM, Boudreau R, et al. Adipokines and the risk of fracture in older adults. J Bone Miner Res 2011;26(7):1568–76.

33. Lee P, Greenfield JR, Seibel MJ, et al. Adequacy of vitamin D replacement in severe deficiency is dependent on body mass index. Am J Med 2009; 122(11):1056–60.

34. Ogunnaike BO, Jones SB, Jones DB, et al. Anesthetic considerations for bariatric surgery. Anesth Analg 2002;95(6):1793–805.

35. Shenkman Z, Shir Y, Brodsky JB. Perioperative management of the obese patient. Br J Anaesth 1993; 70(3):349–59.

36. Jupiter JB, Ring D, Rosen H. The complications and difficulties of management of nonunion in the severely obese. J Orthop Trauma 1995;9(5):363–70.

37. Nielsen KC, Guller U, Steele SM, et al. Influence of obesity on surgical regional anesthesia in the ambulatory setting: an analysis of 9,038 blocks. Anesthesiology 2005;102(1):181–7.

38. Ingrande J, Brodsky JB, Lemmens HJ. Regional anesthesia and obesity. Curr Opin Anaesthesiol 2009;22(5):683–6.

39. Nielson CM, Marshall LM, Adams AL, et al. BMI and fracture risk in older men: the Osteoporotic Fractures in Men Study (MrOS). J Bone Miner Res 2011;26(3):496–502.

40. Cotter JT, Nielsen KC, Guller U, et al. Increased body mass index and ASA physical status IV are risk factors for block failure in ambulatory surgery - an analysis of 9,342 blocks. Can J Anaesth 2004; 51(8):810–6.

41. Edmiston CE, Krepel C, Kelly H, et al. Perioperative antibiotic prophylaxis in the gastric bypass patient: do we achieve therapeutic levels? Surgery 2004; 136(4):738–47.

42. Franco CD, Gloss FJ, Voronov G, et al. Supraclavicular block in the obese population: an analysis of 2020 blocks. Anesth Analg 2006;102(4):1252–4.

43. Eichinger S, Hron G, Bialonczyk C, et al. Overweight, obesity, and the risk of recurrent venous thromboembolism. Arch Intern Med 2008;168(15): 1678–83.

44. Lucena J, Rico A, Vázquez R, et al. Pulmonary embolism and sudden-unexpected death: prospective study on 2477 forensic autopsies performed at the Institute of Legal Medicine in Seville. J Forensic Leg Med 2009;16(4):196–201.

45. Meissner MH, Chandler WL, Elliott JS. Venous thromboembolism in trauma: a local manifestation of systemic hypercoagulability? J Trauma 2003; 54(2):224–31.

46. Memtsoudis SG, Besculides MC, Gaber L, et al. Risk factors for pulmonary embolism after hip and knee arthroplasty: a population-based study. Int Orthop 2009;33(6):1739–45.

47. Blom JW, Doggen CJ, Osanto S, et al. Old and new risk factors for upper extremity deep venous thrombosis. J Thromb Haemost 2005;3(11):2471–8.

48. Porter SE, Graves ML, Qin Z, et al. Operative experience of pelvic fractures in the obese. Obes Surg 2008;18(6):702–8.

49. Porter SE, Russell GV, Dews RC, et al. Complications of acetabular fracture surgery in morbidly obese patients. J Orthop Trauma 2008;22(9): 589–94.

50. Kerkhoffs GM, Servien E, Dunn W, et al. The influence of obesity on the complication rate and outcome of total knee arthroplasty: a meta-analysis and systematic literature review. J Bone Joint Surg Am 2012;94(20):1839–44.

51. Yuan K, Chen HL. Obesity and surgical site infections risk in orthopedics: a meta-analysis. Int J Surg 2013;11(5):383–8.

52. Haley RW, Culver DH, White JW, et al. The nationwide nosocomial infection rate. A new need for vital statistics. Am J Epidemiol 1985; 121(2):159–67.

53. Baldwin KD, Matuszewski PE, Namdari S, et al. Does morbid obesity negatively affect the hospital course of patients undergoing treatment of closed, lower-extremity diaphyseal long-bone fractures? Orthopedics 2011;34(1):18.

54. Green E, Lubahn JD, Evans J. Risk factors, treatment, and outcomes associated with nonunion of the midshaft humerus fracture. J Surg Orthop Adv 2005;14(2):64–72.

55. King AR, Moran SL, Steinmann SP. Humeral nonunion. Hand Clin 2007;23(4):449–56, vi.

56. Strauss EJ, Frank JB, Walsh M, et al. Does obesity influence the outcome after the operative treatment of ankle fractures? J Bone Joint Surg Br 2007;89(6):794–8.

57. Compston JE, Flahive J, Hooven FH, et al. Obesity, health-care utilization, and health-related quality of life after fracture in postmenopausal women: Global Longitudinal Study of Osteoporosis in Women (GLOW). Calcif Tissue Int 2014;94(2): 223–31.

58. Werner BC, Griffin JW, Yang S, et al. Obesity is associated with increased postoperative complications after operative management of proximal humerus fractures. J Shoulder Elbow Surg 2015; 24(4):593–600.

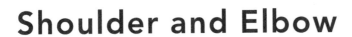

Shoulder and Elbow

Shoulder and Elbow

The Effect of Obesity in Shoulder Arthroplasty Outcomes and Complications

Ivan De Martino, MD[a], Lawrence V. Gulotta, MD[b],*

KEYWORDS

- Total shoulder arthroplasty • Reverse shoulder arthroplasty • Shoulder hemiarthroplasty
- Obesity • Morbid obesity • BMI • Complications • Revision shoulder arthroplasty

---

KEY POINTS

- The effect of obesity on outcomes and complications in shoulder arthroplasty has been recently reported in the literature with different and conflicting results.
- Obesity should be better stratified in classes according to the World Health Organization to better understand its impact on outcomes and complications in shoulder arthroplasty.
- Morbid obesity (body mass index >40 kg/m^2), more than obesity, is associated with a longer operative time, higher complication rate, reoperation rate, and superficial infection.
- Obesity does not have a detrimental effect on functional outcomes. The magnitude of functional improvement in the obese patients, however, can be inferior to that in nonobese patients.
- Obesity and morbid obesity do not increase hospital charges.

INTRODUCTION

Shoulder arthroplasty is an effective operation providing pain relief and improvement of function in patients with end-stage degenerative shoulder disease that is nonresponsive to nonoperative treatments.[1–4] The successful long-term results of shoulder arthroplasty (anatomic, reverse, and hemiarthroplasty) for various indications have previously been reported in the literature.[5–15] Because patients live longer and remain active into later decades of life, the number of shoulder arthroplasties performed in the United States has been increasing over recent years.[7,16] With the increased number of arthroplasties performed and the expanding indications for shoulder arthroplasty, however, the number of revision shoulder arthroplasties is increasing too.[17–26]

To minimize complications and optimize patient outcomes, efforts have been made to identify patient risk factors that are significantly associated with perioperative complications and implant failures.

Obesity has been shown associated with increased rates of complications after orthopedic surgery, such as postoperative infections, intraoperative fractures, and need for revision surgeries.[27–46] According to the World Health Organization (WHO), obesity is defined as a body mass index (BMI) greater than 30 (kg/m^2).[47] The prevalence of obesity is increasing in recent years among adults worldwide, particularly in the United States, where the adult population with a BMI greater than 30 kg/m^2 has been estimated to be 35% and predicted to reach 50% by the year 2030.[48,49]

Disclosure Statement: The authors have nothing to disclose that relates to the subject matter or materials discussed in this article. No funding was received.
[a] Sports and Shoulder Service, Hospital for Special Surgery, Weill Cornell Medical College, 535 East 70th Street, New York, NY 10021, USA; [b] Sports and Shoulder Service, Hospital for Special Surgery, East River Professional Building, 523 East 72nd Street, 6th Floor, New York, NY 10021, USA
* Corresponding author.
E-mail address: gulottal@hss.edu

The relationship between obesity and outcomes and/or complications in lower extremity arthroplasty has been well studied, whereas there has been a paucity of studies examining the effects of obesity on shoulder arthroplasty. The effect of obesity on outcomes and complications in shoulder arthroplasty has been recently reported in the literature with different and conflicting results.[12,40,50–67] These studies are heterogeneous in their study designs, patient cohort sizes, outcomes measures, and follow-up length.[12,40,50–67] There is a lack of studies, however, that have broadly evaluated the existing literature.

This review analyzes the role of obesity on clinical outcomes and complications. Functional outcomes and costs in shoulder arthroplasty are also assessed.

MATERIALS AND METHODS

A review of the literature was performed according to the Preferred Reporting Items for Systematic Reviews and Meta-Analyses guidelines[68] to identify studies reporting outcomes of shoulder arthroplasty in obese patients.

A search of Pubmed, Medline, Embase, and Google Scholar was conducted using various combinations of the keywords, "shoulder", "arthroplasty", "replacement", "obesity", and "weight". No limit was set with regard to the year of publication.

Two independent researchers (the authors, I. De Martino and L.V. Gulotta) scanned all the articles for titles and abstracts. Disagreements were resolved by arbitration, and consensus was reached after discussion. The last search was performed in October 2017. Only articles in English were included. In addition, reference lists of the included articles were manually checked by the authors for missed studies. Ultimately, the search yielded 20 articles deemed relevant.[12,40,50–67]

Of the 20 included articles, 8 were case series in which patients were stratified according their BMI class[12,50–56]; 2 were case series, including only patients with a BMI greater than 40 kg/m^2 (morbidly obese)[40,57]; 9 were analysis of national databases[58–66]; and 1 was a large health care registry analysis.[67]

Effect of Obesity on Clinical Outcomes and Complications

Linberg and colleagues[40] were the first to evaluate outcomes of shoulder arthroplasty in morbidly obese patients. They evaluated 45 shoulder arthroplasties performed for osteoarthritis in patients with a BMI greater than 40 kg/m^2 with a minimum follow-up of 2 years. They found there was significant improvement in pain and function. A longer operative time was reported, however, due to a more challenging surgical exposure and soft tissue management due to the excessive adiposity. There was a higher perioperative complication rate, with 1 significant complication and 5 revisions that led to a higher rate (29%) of unsatisfied patients.

Statz and colleagues[57] performed a similar analysis using the Mayo Clinic Total Joint Registry. They reviewed all primary reverse total shoulder arthroplasties (TSAs) performed on morbidly obese (BMI >40 kg/m^2) patients at their institution from 2005 to 2012 with at least 2 years of follow-up. Of the 41 patients included in their analysis, 2 of them required revision surgery for infection and humeral loosening. The survivorship was 98% at 2 years and 95% at 5 years. They concluded that reverse TSA was a successful procedure in morbidly obese patients with a reasonable complication rate.

Wagner and colleagues,[50] using the same Mayo Clinic Total Joint Registry, investigated the effect of BMI on implant survival and the rate of complications after shoulder arthroplasty. A total of 4567 consecutive shoulder arthroplasties performed from 1970 to 2013 were included in their analysis. The mean BMI of their cohort was 29.7 kg/m^2 (range 14–66 kg/m^2), with 1622 (36%) having a BMI between 30 kg/m^2 and 40 kg/m^2, and 297 patients having a BMI greater than 40 kg/m^2. The investigators found that increasing BMI was associated with an increased risk of a revision surgical procedure, reoperation, superficial infection, and revision for mechanical failure, and it was negatively associated with risk of periprosthetic fracture. Compared with nonobese patients, the risk of reoperation in morbidly obese patients was increased of 46%. This association remained similar when stratified by implant type (hemiarthroplasty, anatomic, or reverse), surgical indication, and glenoid type (metal-backed or all-polyethylene). They found a stronger association between BMI and superficial wound infection, with an increased risk of 82% of any infection in morbidly obese patients relative to nonobese patients. It is clear from this study that increasing BMI is strongly associated with increased rates of postoperative complications and revision surgical procedures.

Similar results were reported by Gupta and colleagues.[56] They analyzed the effect of BMI in 119 patients who had a reverse TSA at their institution with a minimum of 90 days' follow-up. Patients were divided according to their BMI in 3 groups: normal weight (18.5–25 kg/m^2), overweight or mildly obese (25–35 kg/m^2), and moderately or severely obese (>35 kg/m^2). There were 30 normal weight patients, 65 overweight or mildly obese patients, and 24 moderately or severely obese. They found that BMI greater than 35 kg/m^2 was significantly associated with higher overall complication rate and intraoperative blood loss. Patients with BMI less than 25 kg/m^2 had a higher rate of complications too.

Beck and colleagues[52] reported similar results in reverse TSA when analyzing their cohort of patients. They included 76 reverse TSAs performed between 2005 and 2011 and stratified the population by BMI. The complication rate was significantly higher in the obese group (35%) compared with the normal-weight group (4%).

Werner and colleagues[62–64] performed 3 different analyses using the PearlDriver Patient Record Database (www.pearldriver.com; PearlDriver Technologies, Fort Wayne, Indiana). This is a publicly available subscription patient database and contains data derived from a Medicare database with more than 100 million unique patient records from 2005 to 2012. The investigators identified the patients using the *International Classification Disease, Ninth Revision (ICD-9)* diagnoses and procedures or Current Procedural Terminology (CPT) codes. They investigated the patient factors associated with early revision within 1 year after shoulder arthroplasty,[62] the complication rates after shoulder arthroplasty in superobese (BMI >50 kg/m^2) patients[63] and the effect of obesity on postoperative complications after operative management of proximal humerus fractures.[64]

In the first study, the authors evaluated 221,381 patients and found that obesity and morbid obesity were associated with early revision after TSA, hemiarthroplasty, and reverse TSA. Younger age, smoking, and male gender were associated with early revision too.[62]

In the second study, the investigators evaluated 144,239 patients, including 23,864 obese patients; 13,759 morbidly obese patients; and 955 superobese patients. They found that obesity was associated with significantly increased rates of numerous complications after shoulder arthroplasty, including infection, dislocation, component loosening, revision surgery, venous thromboembolism (VTE), and medical complications compared with nonobese patients. Superobesity (BMI >50 kg/m^2) was associated with significantly increased rates of numerous complications, including infection, component loosening, VTE, and medical complications compared with even obese and morbidly obese patients.[63]

In the third study, the investigators evaluated 20,319 patients, including 3391 (16.7%) hemiarthroplasties and 727 (3.6%) TSAs from 2010 to 2014. Within the hemiarthroplasty group, 821 patients (24.2%) were coded as obese. The obese hemiarthroplasty patients had a significantly increased risk of 90-day local and systemic complications and higher rates of postoperative VTE and infection. Within the TSA patients, 256 (35.2%) were coded as obese. The obese TSA patients had also a significantly increased risk of 90-day local and systemic complications and higher rate of infection. The rate of postoperative VTE was not significantly different among obese and nonobese patients.[64]

These studies have several limitations that are inherent to all studies using large administrative database, so clinical significance cannot be determined because outcome measures are not included.

Using the American College of Surgeons National Surgical Quality Improvement (NSQIP) database, Jiang and colleagues[59] compared the 30-day complication profile and hospitalization outcomes after primary TSA among patients with different BMI class. The NSQIP database is a prospectively maintained database that contains perioperative data on randomly assigned patients from more than 480 participating hospitals and offers surveillance of specific clinical outcomes up to the 30th postoperative day, regardless of when a patient was discharged. The investigators analyzed 4267 patients who underwent primary TSA (anatomic and reverse) for shoulder osteoarthritis from 2006 to 2013. Patients were divided according to their BMI in 4 groups: normal (18.5–25 kg/m^2), overweight (25–30 kg/m^2), obesity class I (30–35 kg/m^2), and obesity class II or greater (>35 kg/m^2). There were 738 normal patients, 1463 overweight patients, 1126 class I obese patients and 940 class II obese patients, with obese patients representing 47% of the overall population. The investigators found that there was no association between BMI and 30-day complications after surgery. Greater BMI was associated with longer surgical times.

Using the same NSQIP database, Garcia and colleagues[60] analyzed the effect of metabolic syndrome and obesity on complications after shoulder arthroplasty. Their study population included 4751 patients who received a shoulder arthroplasty from 2005 to 2013. Patients were categorized by BMI in 4 different groups: 2457 nonobese patients, 1235 class I obese patients, 619 class II obese patients, and 440 class III obese patients. The investigators found that class III obese patients had an increased risk of complications and a significantly increased risk of extended length of stay compared with non-obese patients. Metabolic syndrome was not a significant predictor of postoperative complications or extended length of stay.

Similar results were reported by Waterman and colleagues[58] in their study using the NSQIP database. They looked at risk factors for 30-day postoperative complications and mortality. Their study population included 2004 patients. Patients were categorized by BMI in 3 different groups: 1073 (54%) nonobese patients, 760 (38.3%) class I obese patients, 154 (7.7%), and class II or greater obese patients. Obesity was not associated with any specified complications after controlling for other variables.

Griffin and colleagues[61] queried the Nationwide Inpatient Sample database to determine whether morbidly obese patients exhibit greater rates of postoperative in-hospital complications, mortality, or utilization of resources. They analyzed 31,924 patients who received a shoulder arthroplasty from 1998 to 2008. Patients were categorized by BMI in 3 different groups: 29,536 (92.5%) nonobese patients, 1857 (5.7%) obese patients, and 583 (1.8%) morbidly obese patients. A multivariate analysis with logistic regression modeling was performed to compare patients based on their BMI for different outcomes. The investigators found that obese patients tended to have longer hospital stays and increased risk of postoperative respiratory complications and higher costs. There was no association between obesity and increased risk of most complications.

Using the Kaiser Permanente Shoulder Arthroplasty Registry, Anakwenze and colleagues[67] looked at the effect of BMI on postoperative complications. This registry monitors postoperative complications, such as infections, mortality, revisions, readmissions, and reoperations. They included all elective anatomic and reverse TSAs performed between January 2007 and June 2012 in the 2 largest geographic regions (Southern California and Northern California) that participated in the registry. A total of 4630 patients were included, of whom 3483 were anatomic TSAs and 1147 were reverse TSAs. Patients were divided according to their BMI in 5 groups: 872 normal patients, 1670 overweight patients, 1205 class I obese patients, 580 class II obese patients, and 303 class III obese patients. The investigators found that higher BMI was not associated with higher risk of aseptic revision, 1-year mortality, or 3-year mortality. In anatomic TSA model, every increase of 5 kg/m^2 in BMI was marginally associated with a 16% increased risk of readmission within 90 days; however, this was not observed for reverse TSA. In the reverse TSA model, every increase of 5 kg/m^2 in BMI was marginally associated with an increased risk of 3-year deep infection, which was not observed in anatomic TSA (Box 1).

Effect of Obesity on Functional Outcomes

Li and colleagues[53] first investigated the role of obesity on short-term functional outcomes. The investigators compared the functional outcomes and complications in patients who had anatomic TSA. From their prospective shoulder arthroplasty registry, a total of 76 patients who had a TSA between 2009 and 2010 with a minimum follow-up of 2 years were identified. Patients were divided according their BMI in 3 groups: 26 had a normal weight (BMI <25 kg/m^2), 25 were overweight (BMI 25–30 kg/m^2), and 25 were obese (BMI >30 kg/m^2). Shoulder function was assessed with the American Shoulder and Elbow Surgeons (ASES) score, the 36-Item Short Form Health Survey (SF-36), and visual analog scale pain and function scores. The investigators found that obesity did not have a detrimental effect on short-term shoulder function. The overall physical function of obese and overweight patients improved significantly less compared with patients in the normal group. The improvement in the physical SF-36 ranged from 2% to 12% in the obese patients compared with an improvement of 11% to 40% in the normal-weight patients.

Similar results were reported by Morris and colleagues,[54] who investigated the role of obesity on short-term functional outcomes after reverse TSA. The investigators queried their prospective shoulder arthroplasty registry

---

Box 1
Summary of key points for clinical outcomes and complications

- Obesity and morbid obesity are associated with a longer operative time, higher complication rate, reoperation rate, and superficial infection.

- Results from case series are different from results from large national databases.

- Morbid obesity has a detrimental effect on outcomes and complications, more than obesity.

to identify 77 patients who had a reverse TSA between 2004 and 2011 with a minimum follow-up of 2 years. Patients were divided according their BMI in 3 groups: 34 had a normal weight (BMI <25 kg/m²), 21 were overweight (BMI 25–30 kg/m²), and 22 were obese (BMI >30 kg/m²). Shoulder function was assessed with the ASES score, Constant Score, Western Ontario Osteoarthritis Shoulder index, Single Assessment Numeric Evaluation, mobility, and patient satisfaction. The investigators found that the magnitude of change (improvement) from before surgery to final follow-up was almost identical among the 3 BMI groups, with no significant difference in shoulder function scores or mobility. There was no statistical difference in the complication rate either.

Similar results were reported by Pappou and colleagues[12] in patients who had a reverse TSA for indications other than fracture from 2003 to 2010, with a mean of 4 years of follow-up. The investigators compared 21 morbidly obese (BMI >40 kg/m²) patients to 63 nonobese (BMI <30 kg/m²) patients. Shoulder function was assessed with the ASES score, Simple Shoulder Test, visual analog scale pain and function scores, duration of hospital stay, and discharge disposition. There was no statistical difference in the ASES scores and in shoulder motion between morbidly obese patients and nonobese patients. The rate of discharge to rehabilitation facilities, however, rather than home was 6-fold higher for the morbidly obese patients. The investigators found also a significant increase in hospital cost in the morbidly obese population.

Vincent and colleagues[55] analyzed the role of obesity on midterm functional outcomes. They reviewed 310 patients who had a TSA (anatomic and reverse) with a mean follow-up of 5 years (range 3–17 years). Patients were divided according their BMI in 3 groups: 167 were nonobese (BMI <30 kg/m²), 121 were obese (BMI 30–40 kg/m²), and 22 were morbidly obese (BMI >40 kg/m²). Shoulder function was assessed with the ASES score, Shoulder Pain and Disability Index, University of California, Los Angeles rating scale, Constant Score, 12-Item Short Form Health Survey, mobility and radiographic outcomes. They found that obesity did not have a detrimental effect on the improvement in midterm shoulder function except for active external rotation range of motion, possibly due to the morphologic limitation of excessive adiposity. Morbidly obese patients improved significantly less compared with non–morbidly obese patients, as already reported by Li and colleagues.[53]

Poorer functional outcomes in morbidly obese patients were reported by Izquierdo-Fernández and colleagues[51] in the medium term. They analyzed 29 patients who had a reverse TSA and noted a significantly lower ASES score in patients with a BMI greater than 35 kg/m² compared with a BMI lower than 35 kg/m². When the same patient cohort was divided into nonobese (BMI <30 kg/m²) and obese (BMI >30 kg/m²) cohorts, however, statistical difference was found between the 2 groups (**Box 2**).

Obesity and Cost Analysis

Rosas and colleagues[65] evaluated the effect of common medical comorbidities on the reimbursement for different shoulder arthroplasty procedures. They used the Humana private-payer insurance dataset from the PearlDiver Patient Record Database (www.pearldiverinc.com; Pearl-Diver Technologies, Fort Wayne, Indiana) for analysis. A total of 23,879 patients were identified using *ICD-9* and CPT codes. They analyzed the effect of comorbidities on the reimbursement charges for the day of surgery, 90-day global period, and 90-day period, excluding the initial surgical day. The investigators found that obesity and morbid obesity did not have a significant effect on initial day of surgery reimbursement cost, 90-day cost, and 89-day cost (90-day period excluding the initial surgical day) compared with the annual mean reimbursement used as control.

Davis and colleagues[66] evaluated the effect of arthritic etiology, multiple medical comorbidities, and patient and hospital demographics on total in-hospital charges by a multivariate analysis using the Nationwide Inpatient Sample database. This database was created as part of the Healthcare Cost and Utilization Project and includes more than 7 million hospital stays at more than 1000 hospitals (rural, urban, and academic), representing a 20% sample of hospitals in the United States. The investigators queried

---

Box 2
Summary of key points for functional outcomes

- Obesity does not have a detrimental effect on functional outcomes.

- The magnitude of functional improvement in the obese patients can be inferior to the nonobese patients.

- Improvement in range of motion can be limited due to the morphologic limitation of excessive adiposity.

Box 3
Summary of key point for cost analysis

- Obesity and morbid obesity do not increase hospital charges from large national databases.

---

this database to evaluate total hospital charges for 52,982 patients who had shoulder arthroplasty from 1993 to 2010. Obesity was found to not increase hospital charges significantly, whether or not obese patients were diabetic (**Box 3**).

SUMMARY

The effect of obesity on outcomes and complications in shoulder arthroplasty has been recently reported in the literature with different and conflicting results.[12,40,50–67] On analysis of the data in the current literature, some considerations can be made despite the heterogeneity of the study designs, patient cohort sizes, outcomes measures, and follow-up length. Obese patients may have outcomes similar to normal-weight and overweight patients. When the obese patient population is better stratified according to their BMI, in morbidly obese and superobese patients, however, the effect of BMI on outcomes and complications is more evident. Half of the studies (10 of 20) considered for this review were from large databases and linked to several limitations that are inherent to all studies using these data repositories. As such, clinical significance cannot be determined because outcome measures are not included. Further research is needed to better define the effects of obesity on outcomes in shoulder arthroplasty. The current literature indicates, however, that the presence of obesity does not increase costs of care significantly over nonobese patients.

REFERENCES

1. Chalmers PN, Gupta AK, Rahman Z, et al. Predictors of early complications of total shoulder arthroplasty. J Arthroplasty 2014;29:856–60.
2. Deshmukh AV, Koris M, Zurakowski D, et al. Total shoulder arthroplasty: long-term survivorship, functional outcome, and quality of life. J Shoulder Elbow Surg 2005;14:471–9.
3. Montoya F, Magosch P, Scheiderer B, et al. Midterm results of a total shoulder prosthesis fixed with a cementless glenoid component. J Shoulder Elbow Surg 2013;22:628–35.
4. Torchia ME, Cofield RH, Settergren CR. Total shoulder arthroplasty with the Neer prosthesis: long-term results. J Shoulder Elbow Surg 1997;6: 495–505.
5. Carter MJ, Mikuls TR, Nayak C, et al. Impact of total shoulder arthroplasty on generic and shoulder-specific healthrelated quality-of-life measures: a systematic literature review and meta-analysis. J Bone Joint Surg Am 2012;94:e127.
6. Denard PJ, Raiss P, Sowa B, et al. Mid- to long-term follow-up of total shoulder arthroplasty using a keeled glenoid in young adults with primary glenohumeral arthritis. J Shoulder Elbow Surg 2013;22: 894–900.
7. Dillon MT, Inacio MC, Burke MF, et al. Shoulder arthroplasty in patients 59 years of age and younger. J Shoulder Elbow Surg 2013;22:1338–44.
8. Ek ET, Neukom L, Catanzaro S, et al. Reverse total shoulder arthroplasty for massive irreparable rotator cuff tears in patients younger than 65 years old: results after five to fifteen years. J Shoulder Elbow Surg 2013;22:1199–208.
9. Favard L, Katz D, Colmar M, et al. Total shoulder arthroplastydarthroplasty for glenohumeral arthropathies: results and complications after a minimum follow-up of 8 years according to the type of arthroplasty and etiology. Orthop Traumatol Surg Res 2012;98(Suppl 4):S41–7.
10. Griffin JW, Hadeed MM, Novicoff WM, et al. Patient age is a factor in early outcomes after shoulder arthroplasty. J Shoulder Elbow Surg 2014;23: 1867–71.
11. Muh SJ, Streit JJ, Wanner JP, et al. Early follow-up of reverse total shoulder arthroplasty in patients sixty years of age or younger. J Bone Joint Surg Am 2013;95:1877–83.
12. Pappou I, Virani NA, Clark R, et al. Outcomes and Costs of reverse shoulder arthroplasty in the morbidly obese: a case control study. J Bone Joint Surg Am 2014;96:1169–76.
13. Shields E, Iannuzzi JC, Thorsness R, et al. Perioperative complications after hemiarthroplasty and total shoulder arthroplasty are equivalent. J Shoulder Elbow Surg 2014;23:1449–53.
14. Sperling JW, Cofield RH, Rowland CM. Minimum fifteen-year follow-up of Neer hemiarthroplasty and total shoulder arthroplasty in patients aged fifty years or younger. J Shoulder Elbow Surg 2004;13:604–13.
15. Young SW, Zhu M, Walker CG, et al. Comparison of functional outcomes of reverse shoulder arthroplasty with those of hemiarthroplasty in the treatment of cuff-tear arthropathy: a matched-pair analysis. J Bone Joint Surg Am 2013;95:910–5.
16. Kim SH, Wise BL, Zhang Y, et al. Increasing incidence of shoulder arthroplasty in the United States. J Bone Joint Surg Am 2011;93:2249–54.

17. Antuna SA, Sperling JW, Cofield RH, et al. Glenoid revision surgery after total shoulder arthroplasty. J Shoulder Elbow Surg 2001;10:217–24.
18. Chalmers PN, Rahman Z, Romeo AA, et al. Early dislocation after reverse total shoulder arthroplasty. J Shoulder Elbow Surg 2014;23:737–44.
19. Farng E, Zingmond D, Krenek L, et al. Factors predicting complication rates after primary shoulder arthroplasty. J Shoulder Elbow Surg 2011;20:557–63.
20. Farshad M, Grogli M, Catanzaro S, et al. Revision of reversed total shoulder arthroplasty. Indications and outcome. BMC Musculoskelet Disord 2012;13:160.
21. Fevang BT, Lie SA, Havelin LI, et al. Risk factors for revision after shoulder arthroplasty: 1,825 shoulder arthroplasties from the Norwegian Arthroplasty Register. Acta Orthop 2009;80:83–91.
22. Fox TJ, Cil A, Sperling JW, et al. Survival of the glenoid component in shoulder arthroplasty. J Shoulder Elbow Surg 2009;18:859–63.
23. Rasmussen JV. Outcome and risk of revision following shoulder replacement in patients with glenohumeral osteoarthritis. Acta Orthop Suppl 2014;85:1–23.
24. Rasmussen JV, Polk A, Brorson S, et al. Patient-reported outcome and risk of revision after shoulder replacement for osteoarthritis. 1,209 cases from the Danish shoulder arthroplasty registry, 2006-2010. Acta Orthop 2014;85:117–22.
25. Sajadi KR, Kwon YW, Zuckerman JD. Revision shoulder arthroplasty: an analysis of indications and outcomes. J Shoulder Elbow Surg 2010;19:308–13.
26. Singh JA, Sperling JW, Cofield RH. Revision surgery following total shoulder arthroplasty: analysis of 2588 shoulders over three decades (1976 to 2008). J Bone Joint Surg Br 2011;93:1513–7.
27. Amin AK, Clayton RA, Patton JT, et al. Total knee replacement in morbidly obese patients. Results of a prospective, matched study. J Bone Joint Surg Br 2006;88:1321–6.
28. Amin AK, Patton JT, Cook RE, et al. Does obesity influence the clinical outcome at five years following total knee replacement for osteoarthritis? J Bone Joint Surg Br 2006;88:335–40.
29. Arsoy D, Woodcock JA, Lewallen DG, et al. Outcomes and complications following total hip arthroplasty in the super-obese patient, BMI >50. J Arthroplasty 2014;29:1899–905.
30. Bozic KJ, Lau E, Kurtz S, et al. Patient-related risk factors for postoperative mortality and periprosthetic joint infection in medicare patients undergoing TKA. Clin Orthop Relat Res 2012;470:130–7.
31. Bozic KJ, Lau E, Kurtz S, et al. Patient-related risk factors for periprosthetic joint infection and postoperative mortality following total hip arthroplasty in Medicare patients. J Bone Joint Surg Am 2012;94:794–800.
32. Dowsey MM, Liew D, Choong PF. Economic burden of obesity in primary total knee arthroplasty. Arthritis Care Res (Hoboken) 2011;63:1375–81.
33. Foran JR, Mont MA, Etienne G, et al. The outcome of total knee arthroplasty in obese patients. J Bone Joint Surg Am 2004;86-A:1609–15.
34. Griffin FM, Scuderi GR, Insall JN, et al. Total knee arthroplasty in patients who were obese with 10 years followup. Clin Orthop Relat Res 1998;356:28–33.
35. Jaberi FM, Parvizi J, Haytmanek CT, et al. Procrastination of wound drainage and malnutrition affect the outcome of joint arthroplasty. Clin Orthop Relat Res 2008;466:1368–71.
36. Jain NB, Guller U, Pietrobon R, et al. Comorbidities increase complication rates in patients having arthroplasty. Clin Orthop Relat Res 2005;435:232–8.
37. Jämsen E, Nevalainen P, Eskelinen A, et al. Obesity, diabetes, and preoperative hyperglycemia as predictors of periprosthetic joint infection: a single-center analysis of 7181 primary hip and knee replacements for osteoarthritis. J Bone Joint Surg Am 2012;94:e101.
38. Kamath AF, McAuliffe CL, Baldwin KD, et al. Unplanned admission to the intensive care unit after total hip arthroplasty. J Arthroplasty 2012;27:1027–32.e1-2.
39. Kerkhoffs GM, Servien E, Dunn W, et al. The influence of obesity on the complication rate and outcome of total knee arthroplasty: a meta-analysis and systematic literature review. J Bone Joint Surg Am 2012;94:1839–44.
40. Linberg CJ, Sperling JW, Schleck CD, et al. Shoulder arthroplasty in morbidly obese patients. J Shoulder Elbow Surg 2009;18:903–6.
41. Namba RS, Paxton L, Fithian DC, et al. Obesity and perioperative morbidity in total hip and total knee arthroplasty patients. J Arthroplasty 2005;20:46–50.
42. Schwarzkopf R, Thompson SL, Adwar SJ, et al. Postoperative complication rates in the "super-obese" hip and knee arthroplasty population. J Arthroplasty 2012;27:397–401.
43. Silber JH, Rosenbaum PR, Kelz RR, et al. Medical and financial risks associated with surgery in the elderly obese. Ann Surg 2012;256:79–86.
44. Spicer DD, Pomeroy DL, Badenhausen WE, et al. Body mass index as a predictor of outcome in total knee replacement. Int Orthop 2001;25:246–9.
45. Stern SH, Insall JN. Total knee arthroplasty in obese patients. J Bone Joint Surg Am 1990;72:1400–4.
46. Wade FA, Parvizi J, Sharkey PF, et al. Femoral perforation complicating contemporary uncemented hip arthroplasty. J Arthroplasty 2006;21:452–5.

47. World Health Organization. Global Database on Body Mass Index. Available at: http://apps.who.int/bmi/index.jsp?introPage=intro_3.html. Accessed October 21, 2017.

48. Abdel MP, Ast MP, Lee YY, et al. All-cause in-hospital complications and urinary tract infections increased in obese patients undergoing total knee arthroplasty. J Arthroplasty 2014;29: 1430–4.

49. Wang Y, Beydoun MA, Liang L, et al. Will all Americans become overweight or obese? estimating the progression and cost of the US obesity epidemic. Obesity (Silver Spring) 2008; 16:2323–30.

50. Wagner ER, Houdek MT, Schleck C, et al. Increasing body mass index is associated with worse outcomes after shoulder arthroplasty. J Bone Joint Surg Am 2017;99:929–37.

51. Izquierdo-Fernández A, Minarro JC, Carpintero-Lluch R, et al. Reverse shoulder arthroplasty in obese patients: analysis of functionality in the medium-term. Arch Orthop Trauma Surg 2017. https://doi.org/10.1007/s00402-017-2816-6.

52. Beck JD, Irgit KS, Andreychik CM, et al. Reverse total shoulder arthroplasty in obese patients. J Hand Surg Am 2013;38(5):965–70.

53. Li X, Williams PN, Nguyen JT, et al. Functional outcomes after total shoulder arthroplasty in obese patients. J Bone Joint Surg Am 2013;95: e160.

54. Morris BJ, Haigler RE, Cochran JM, et al. Obesity has minimal impact on short-term functional scores after reverse shoulder arthroplasty for rotator cuff tear arthropathy. Am J Orthop (Belle Mead NJ) 2016;45(4):E180–6.

55. Vincent HK, Struk AM, Reed A, et al. Mid-term shoulder functional and quality of life outcomes after shoulder replacement in obese patients. Springerplus 2016;5(1):1929.

56. Gupta AK, Chalmers PN, Rahman Z, et al. Reverse total shoulder arthroplasty in patients of varying body mass index. J Shoulder Elbow Surg 2014; 23(1):35–42.

57. Statz JM, Wagner ER, Houdek MT, et al. Outcomes of primary reverse shoulder arthroplasty in patients with morbid obesity. J Shoulder Elbow Surg 2016; 25(7):e191–8.

58. Waterman BR, Dunn JC, Bader J, et al. Thirty-day morbidity and mortality after elective total shoulder arthroplasty: patient-based and surgical risk factors. J Shoulder Elbow Surg 2015;24(1):24–30.

59. Jiang JJ, Somogyi JR, Patel PB, et al. Obesity is not associated with increased short-term complications after primary total shoulder arthroplasty. Clin Orthop Relat Res 2016;474(3):787–95.

60. Garcia GH, Fu MC, Webb ML, et al. Effect of metabolic syndrome and obesity on complications after shoulder arthroplasty. Orthopedics 2016;39(5): 309–16.

61. Griffin JW, Novicoff WM, Browne JA, et al. Morbid obesity in total shoulder arthroplasty: risk, outcomes, and cost analysis. J Shoulder Elbow Surg 2014;23(10):1444–8.

62. Werner BC, Burrus MT, Begho I, et al. Early revision within 1 year after shoulder arthroplasty: patient factors and etiology. J Shoulder Elbow Surg 2015; 24(12):e323–30.

63. Werner BC, Burrus MT, Browne JA, et al. Superobesity (body mass index >50 kg/m2) and complications after total shoulder arthroplasty: an incremental effect of increasing body mass index. J Shoulder Elbow Surg 2015;24(12):1868–75.

64. Werner BC, Griffin JW, Yang S, et al. Obesity is associated with increased postoperative complications after operative management of proximal humerus fractures. J Shoulder Elbow Surg 2015; 24(4):593–600.

65. Rosas S, Sabeh KG, Buller LT, et al. Comorbidity effects on shoulder arthroplasty costs analysis of a nationwide private payer insurance data set. J Shoulder Elbow Surg 2017;26(7):e216–21.

66. Davis DE, Paxton ES, Maltenfort M, et al. Factors affecting hospital charges after total shoulder arthroplasty: an evaluation of the National Inpatient Sample database. J Shoulder Elbow Surg 2014; 23(12):1860–6.

67. Anakwenze O, Fokin A, Chocas M, et al. Complications in total shoulder and reverse total shoulder arthroplasty by body mass index. J Shoulder Elbow Surg 2017;26(7):1230–7.

68. Moher D, Liberati A, Tetzlaff J, et al, PRISMA Group. Preferred reporting items for systematic reviews and meta-analyses: the PRISMA statement. Ann Intern Med 2009;151:264–9.

The Influence of Obesity on Total Elbow Arthroplasty

Mark E. Morrey, MD*, Mario Hevesi, MD

KEYWORDS

- Obesity • BMI • WHO class III obesity • Total elbow arthroplasty • TEA survivorship
- TEA complications

KEY POINTS

- Total elbow arthroplasty (TEA) indications have changed markedly in the past decade to address the sequalae of trauma rather than inflammatory conditions.
- Obesity has risen markedly over the same time frame and is a national health epidemic, with consequences including increased fractures of long bones and decreased bone densities when controlled for body mass.
- Results of TEA in the obese have shown higher complication and failure rates.
- Risk for early failure should be discussed with patients seeking TEA.
- Patients with a body mass index of greater than 40 corresponding to World Health Organization class III obesity have markedly increased rates of complications and failure rates over other classes of obesity.

INTRODUCTION

Total elbow arthroplasty (TEA) has been used for more than decades to treat several pathologic conditions about the elbow. Over the years, TEA has become more prevalent with an expansion of the indications for its use and an evolution of implant design. According to 1 study, the number of primary procedures from 1993 to 2007 increased 248% and the revision procedures increased by 500% in the same period. Annual volume growth rates were projected to increase 6.4% for primary TEA and 12.8% for revisions.[1] Historically, the primary indication for TEA was rheumatoid arthritis. In a recent analysis of data from the authors' institution, however, the proportion of TEA performed for inflammatory conditions has fallen with a proportional rise in procedures done for the sequelae of trauma (**Fig. 1**).[2] Population-based registry data around the world also confirm a similar trend.[3–5]

Disturbingly, although the trend for TEA has increased in those with posttraumatic conditions, body mass index (BMI) has also increased markedly in the same time frame. The World Health Organization (WHO), recognizing this alarming trend, set up 3 classes of BMI in 1995[6] and then further refined these classes in 2000[7] and 2004.[8] The class cutoff points were based principally on the link between obesity and mortality figures and include those listed in **Table 1**.

According to these guidelines, in the United States, approximately 38% of adults are obese[9] and approximately 8% of adults are morbidly obese (BMI ≥40.0).[9] Data from the National Bureau of Economic Research has shown the fastest growing class of obesity to be those with BMIs over 40, which correspond with WHO class III morbid obesity compared with groups with lower BMIs (**Fig. 2**).[10]

The trend in rising BMIs, especially at the higher levels, is alarming because there is a

Department of Orthopaedic Surgery, Mayo Clinic, Gonda 14, 200 First Street Southwest, Rochester, MN 55905, USA
* Corresponding author.
E-mail address: morrey.mark@mayo.edu

Orthop Clin N Am 49 (2018) 361–370
https://doi.org/10.1016/j.ocl.2018.02.009

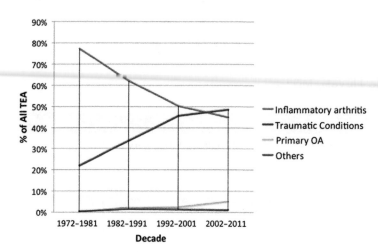

Fig. 1. TEA indications have changed dramatically over the past 4 decades, with the largest proportion of TEA done for traumatic conditions either acutely or due to the sequelae of trauma. OA, osteoarthritis.

linear relationship between obesity and systemic diseases, including coronary heart disease, hypertension, diabetes, gall bladder disease, cancer, and osteoarthritis.[11] With regard to osteoarthritis, a relationship exists for even non–weight-bearing joints, such as the hands.[7] There is a growing body of research linking obesity to a proinflammatory state, which potentiates osteoarthritis through factors, such as leptin and adiponectin, and independent of increased loads across these non–weight-bearing joints.[12–14]

Not only are there known systemic health problems associated with obesity but also obese patients are far more likely to sustain trauma and comminuted fractures, even at low velocity, at the ends of long bones leading to operative intervention.[15] One cross-sectional study of the rates of medically attended injury among adults in the United States showed that the odds of sustaining trauma were 15% (BMI 25–30) to 48% (BMI ≥40) higher among those with excess weight.[16] This may be due to a relative decrease in bone mineral density in obese patients; however, this relationship is conflicting.[17–21] Although obese and overweight adolescents seem to have higher overall bone mineral content than normal-weight counterparts, this effect is reversed when

Table 1
Summary of World Health Organization classes of obesity

Classification	Body Mass Index (kg/m²)	
	Principal Cutoff Points	Additional Cutoff Points
Underweight	<18.50	<18.50
Severe thinness	<16.00	<16.00
Moderate thinness	16.00–16.99	16.00–16.99
Mild thinness	17.00–18.49	17.00–18.49
Normal range	18.50–24.99	18.50–22.99 23.00–24.99
Overweight	≥25.00	≥25.00
Preobese	25.00–29.99	25.00–27.49 27.50–29.99
Obese	≥30.00	≥30.00
Obese class I	30.00–34.99	30.00–32.49 32.50–34.99
Obese class II	35.00–39.99	35.00–37.49 37.50–39.99
Obese class III	≥40.00	≥40.00

From World Health Organization (WHO). Global Database on Body Mass Index. BMI Classification. Available at: http://apps.who.int/bmi/index.jsp?introPage=intro_3.html. Accessed February 9, 2018; with permission.

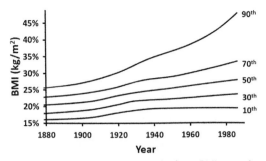

Fig. 2. Those patients with the highest BMIs are the fastest growing group over the past century. (*Data from* Ruhm CJ. Current and future prevalence of obesity and severe obesity in the United States. Cambridge (MA): The National Bureau of Economic Research; 2007.)

controlled for total body mass.[22] Thus, the overall increased bone density in obese patients may not be adequate to overcome the markedly increased forces that are generated during a fall on the upper extremity, leading to comminuted fractures necessitating fixation or TEA. Subsequent falls also put the prosthesis at significant risk for periprosthetic fracture and revision surgery (Fig. 3).[23]

The association between the outcomes, complications, and implant failure after joint replacement arthroplasty in obese patients has also been increasingly recognized in other joints.[23–43] Although country-wide registries might be helpful for elucidating this link further, unfortunately a recent review shows that information about BMI and WHO classes is not routinely collected for the elbow.[44] Even though the link between increased complication rates, worse outcomes, and failure rates due to obesity has been established in the lower extremity, there are far fewer studies specifically examining obesity and TEA. With the growing number of TEAs performed for posttraumatic conditions, parallel increases in obesity for these indications this relationship merit further investigation. Posttraumatic conditions have independently been shown less durable over time compared with those performed for inflammatory conditions in most long-term population studies.[2,3,5] Two primary concerns with TEA have been early loosening and wear of the polyethylene bushings. In the authors' recent analysis, approximately 16% of TEAs done over 20 years were revised for mechanical failure.[45–52] Although only approximately 3%, were revised for bushing wear, as many as 20% showed radiographic evidence of wear.[2] Furthermore, not only has the number of TEAs

performed for inflammatory arthritis decreased but also these patients typically have lower BMIs compared with patients who are undergoing TEA for traumatic or posttraumatic conditions (Table 2).

If there is a negative synergistic effect in the obese population, the combination may well further negatively influence complications and long-term survivorship of the implants. This postulate arises from 2 key observations:

1. Increased body habitus can lead to increased mechanical loads across the elbow joint. In particular, torsional forces are increased proportionally to the weight of the arm in the most everyday activities to place the arm in space. Theoretically this has the potential to (a) accelerate wear and (b) because forces are transmitted to the bone cement and implant cement interfaces, implant loosening.
2. Patients may have an increased risk of wound healing and infection complications due to their thick layer of poorly vascularized adipose tissue, attenuated immune systems, and proinflammatory states.

TOTAL ELBOW ARTHROPLASTY AND OBESITY
Complications of Obesity and Total Elbow Arthroplasty

In studies examining the effect of obesity on TEA, the risk for complications are increased in nearly all the studies examined (Table 3).

In 1 large study of more than 6000 patients with distal humerus fractures, of whom 2700 received a TEA, there was a significantly increased risk of 90-day local and systemic operative and medical complications in obese patients.[53] One of the most feared complications, infection, was more than triple compared with nonobese patients. Although this study did not examine revision rates due to the 90-day follow-up, other studies have shown that not only obese TEA patients have increased risk of major and minor complications, including a 4-times higher medical complication rate, but also these same patients have significantly increased revision rates with implant removal compared with nonobese patients.[54] Other studies have shown similar data with worse outcomes. For example, in midterm results of the Discovery implant in 51 patients, obesity was a major risk factor for infection.[55] In another study of 723 elbows specifically examining the effect of obesity on outcomes, perioperative mortality rates and complications were comparable

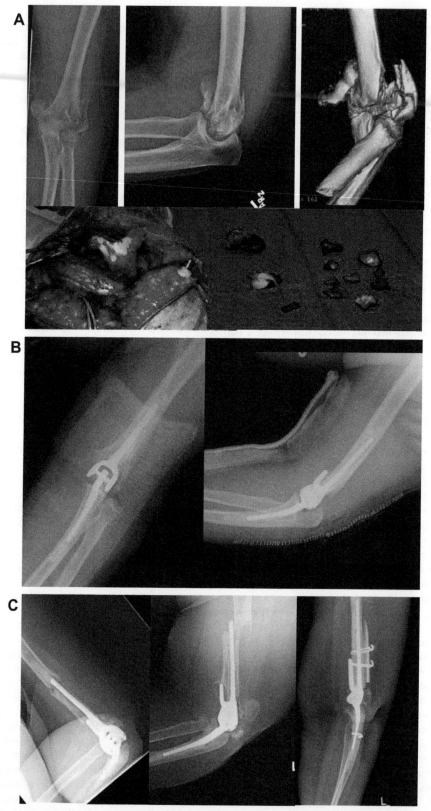

Fig. 3. (*A*) A distal humeral fracture in a patient with a BMI of 48 after a low-energy fall with a severely comminuted articular shear fracture and lateral column fracture. (*B*) The postoperative TEA. (*C*) The same patient after subsequent low-energy trauma leading to a periprosthetic fracture and revision TEA with strut grafting.

Table 2
Patient demographics highlighting body mass index in association with different primary diagnosis in 1299 total elbow arthroplasties

	Inflammatory Arthritis	Posttraumatic Osteoarthritis	Acute Fracture	Other Reasons
BMI (kg/m^2)	25.5 ± 5.7	28.1 ± 6.1	27.7 ± 6.6	28.2 ± 8.7
% BMI over 30	16.5	32.7	29.6	29.2
% BMI over 40	3.2	5.5	8.1	12.5

between nonobese and obese patients, except for extensor mechanism dysfunction and the development of heterotrophic ossification, both of which were greater in obese patients.[56] The reason for triceps disruption is unclear, but a link between the larger forces generated across the elbow in obese patients and greater stress to healing repairs could be postulated. Heterotopic ossification (HO) seems to have a more clear association. It has been shown that obesity is associated with a chronic low-grade inflammatory process that may act as a trigger for the pathogenesis of HO, possibly via increased levels of leptin in obese patients.[57–63] Surprisingly, infection rates were not higher in this cohort of patients.

Survivorship of Total Elbow Arthroplasty in Obese Patients

Several studies have explored the survivorship of various prostheses after TEA, and the general survival rates have been reported to be lower than that for hip and knee arthroplasty, with a wide survivorship ranging from 81% to 90% at 10 years.[3–5,64] Furthermore, like the hip and knee, obesity seems to play a factor in revision surgery in that TEA survivorship depends not only on the primary diagnosis for which elbow replacement is indicated[3,65,66] but also on a patient's BMI.[2,56] Bagdadi and colleagues,[56] in the only study examining long-term outcomes for obesity and TEA, showed in their study of 723 elbows that 118 revisions (16%) were performed overall. The survival free of revision for nonobese patients was 86% compared with only 70% in obese patients (P<.05). Mechanical failures were much higher in this study, with a 10-year survival rate of 88% (95% CI [confidence interval], 84%–91%) in nonobese patients compared with 72% (95% CI, 61%–81%) in obese patients (P<.05). The higher classes of obesity fared more poorly, with higher risks of revision for any reason compared with nonobese patients, with hazard ratios above 3.[56]

CONTEMPORARY RESULTS OF TOTAL ELBOW ARTHROPLASTY IN THE OBESE PATIENT
Complications of Obesity in Total Elbow Arthroplasty Patients in Contemporary Practice

In a recent analysis of the authors' total joint database, a significantly increased risk of complications was found for patients with WHO class III obesity compared with patients with lower and normal BMIs. This analysis included 548 TEAs performed with contemporary operative techniques and implants over the past 15 years. The study cohort included 158 men and 390 women, with a mean age of 61.1 years (range 21–95) at the time of the surgery. Height and weight at the time of the surgery were used to calculate BMI, which was 27.6 (range 11.6–59.7) on average. There were 384 (70%) patients with a normal BMI, 97 (18%) patients with class I, 40 (7%) patients with class II, and 27 (5%) patients with class III obesity. Overall, 30% of patients were classified as obese, which is lower than the national average. After analysis of the complications, there was found a greater risk of fractures (44% vs 14%), decreased motion (15% vs 8%), HO (11% vs 5%), loosening (26% vs 12%), vascular complications (15% vs 6%), and extensor mechanism failures (7% vs 2%) in patients with WHO class III obesity. Complications were expanded from the authors' previous analysis but again included an increased risk of HO and extensor tendon insufficiencies. Surprisingly no significant differences were found in the rate of superficial or deep infection or wound healing problems. Perhaps the most surprising complication was intraoperative and postoperative fracture, which occurred 4 times more often in obese patients. This may be a result of challenging exposures and greater levering of soft tissue envelopes coupled with an increased propensity for trauma and relative decreased bone mineralization, as previously noted in other investigations.

Loosening was twice as likely in this group, again perhaps because of the greater stress

Table 3
Studies examining obesity and total elbow arthroplasty

Study	Years	No. of Patients	Body Mass Index Classes	Follow-up	Summary
Griffin et al,[54] 2015	2005–2011	7580	<30 30–40 >40	2 y	1030 of 7580 patients (14%) were obese (BMI >30) and 611 patients (8%) were morbidly obese (BMI >40). The obese TEA patients had increased risk of 90-d major and minor complications. Medical complications were higher in obese patients (16.7%) compared with the nonobese cohort (4.7%). The rate of postoperative venous thromboembolism was higher in obese patients (2.2%) vs nonobese patients (0.7%). Rate of postoperative stiffness was similar between groups. Infection rates were higher in obese patients. A significant difference in implant removal at 6 mo and 1 y in morbidly obese patients compared with normal-weight counterparts.
Werner et al,[53] 2015	2005–2011	6928	<30 >30	90 d	Of the included cohort, 2713 had TEA procedures. Obese TEA patients had increased risk of 90-d local (odds ratio, 2.6; $P<.0001$) and systemic (odds ratio, 4.4; $P<.0001$) complications. The rates of postoperative infection, venous thromboembolism, and medical complications were higher in the obese TEA cohort.
Large et al,[55] 2014	2008–2011	51	BMI classes not recorded	40.6 mo mean follow-up	Medium-term results of the Discovery elbow. 4/51 TEAs had periprosthetic infection occurred resulting in failure. A statistically significant association between infection and increased BMI was found ($P = .0268$).
Baghdadi et al,[56] 2014	1987–2006	723	<30 >30	5.8 y median f/u	10-y survival rate for TEA was 86% (95% CI, 82%–89%) in nonobese patients compared with 70% (95% CI, 60%–79%) in obese patients ($P<.05$). 10-y survival rate for TEA revision for mechanical failure was 88% (95% CI, 84%–91%) in nonobese patients compared with 72% (95% CI, 61%–81%) in obese patients ($P<.05$). Severely obese patients (those with a BMI of 35 to <40 kg/m^2) had a significantly higher risk of TEA revision for any reason (hazard ratio, 3.08 [95% CI, 1.61–5.45]; $P<.05$) and mechanical failure (hazard ratio, 3.10 [95% CI, 1.47–5.89]; $P<.05$) compared with nonobese patients.

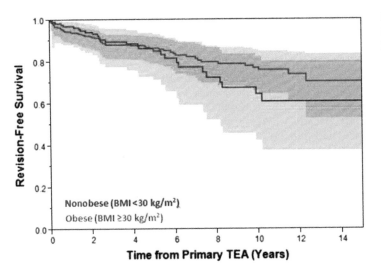

Fig. 4. Revision-free survival comparing obese and nonobese patients with 95% CIs.

across the bone cement interfaces. Nevertheless, these complications were only seen with a BMI over 40 or WHO class III obesity, which may represent a critical threshold for most of the complications observed. The authors are currently investigating whether a critical inflection point truly exists at this cutoff point.

Survivorship of Total Elbow Arthroplasty in Obese Patients in Contemporary Practice

Similar to the complication rates, WHO class III obesity was associated with a significant increase in revision rates over time (revision was defined as removal or exchange of at least 1 component of the TEA and this included 1 one or a combination of humeral, ulnar, and polyethylene-bearing components). Kaplan-Meier survival curves were used to estimate the cumulative risk of revision with the end point set as the date of revision or removal of any prosthesis for any of the previously identified BMI classes. Overall survival up to 14 years was 75%, which has been similar to prior studies, and there was a clear divergence in obese and nonobese patients (**Fig. 4**).

When stratifying into the various classes, however, WHO class III patients again showed worse survivorship compared with the other classes dropping to a mere 35% survivorship at 8 years (**Fig. 5**).

Although WHO class II was also worse, showing 65% survivorship at 10 years, this relationship was not statistically significant. Again, BMIs of 40 or greater seem to play a major role not only in complications but

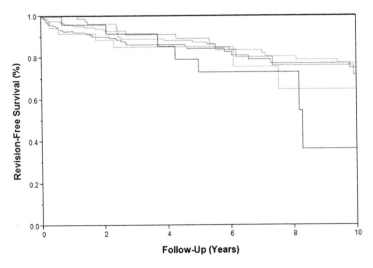

Fig. 5. Revision-free survival separated by BMI class (red: BMI <18.5; green: BMI 18.5–25; blue: BMI 25–30; orange: BMI 30–35; light blue: BMI 35–40; and purple: BMI 40+.).

also on implant survival and may represent a cutoff point above which TEA is unsafe to perform.

SUMMARY

TEA has undergone a significant evolution in indications and outcomes in the last decade. Although rheumatoid patients once had the overwhelming number of TEAs, now TEAs for the sequelae of trauma predominate. Furthermore, as obesity has mirrored the increase in the posttraumatic population, TEA complications have increased whereas the durability of implants under these loads has decreased. Solutions are urgently needed to address the complications and revision burden related to posttraumatic deformity and obesity.

REFERENCES

1. Day JS, Lau E, Ong KL, et al. Prevalence and projections of total shoulder and elbow arthroplasty in the United States to 2015. J Shoulder Elbow Surg 2010;19(8):1115–20.
2. Jo S, Morrey B, Sanchez-Sotelo J, et al. The risk of revision surgery after primary total elbow arthroplasty: a review of 1,261 elbows over four decades. In: AAOS Annual meeting 2015 Proceedings. Paper presented at: Sands Expo and Convention Center. Las Vegas (NV), March 24–28, 2015.
3. Fevang B-TS, Lie SA, Havelin LI, et al. Results after 562 total elbow replacements: a report from the Norwegian Arthroplasty Register. J Shoulder Elbow Surg 2009;18(3):449–56.
4. Jenkins PJ, Watts AC, Norwood T, et al. Total elbow replacement: outcome of 1,146 arthroplasties from the Scottish Arthroplasty Project. Acta Orthop 2013;84(2):119–23.
5. Skytta ET, Eskelinen A, Paavolainen P, et al. Total elbow arthroplasty in rheumatoid arthritis: a population-based study from the Finnish Arthroplasty Register. Acta Orthop 2009;80(4):472–7.
6. WHO. Physical status: the use and interpretation of anthropometry. Report of a WHO Expert Committee. Geneva (Switzerland): World Health Organization; 1995.
7. WHO. Obesity: preventing and managing the global epidemic. Geneva (Switzerland): World Health Organization; 2000.
8. WHO. Appropriate body-mass index for Asian populations and its implications for policy and intervention strategies. Lancet 2004;363(9403):157–63.
9. CDC. National Health and Nutrition Examination Survey. 2013-14. Available at: https://wwwn.cdc.gov/ncha/nhanes/continuousnhanes/faq.aspx?BeginYear=2013. Accessed August 23, 2017.
10. Ruhm C. Current and future prevalence of obesity and severe obesity in the united states. NBER working paper series. 2007. Available at: http://www.nber.org/papers/w13181. Accessed August 23, 2017.
11. World Health Organization. Global database on body mass index. Geneva (Switzerland): World Health Organization; 2017.
12. Aspden RM. Obesity punches above its weight in osteoarthritis. Nature reviews. Rheumatology 2011;7(1):65–8.
13. Berenbaum F, Eymard F, Houard X. Osteoarthritis, inflammation and obesity. Curr Opin Rheumatol 2013;25(1):114–8.
14. Conde J, Scotece M, Lopez V, et al. Adipokines: novel players in rheumatic diseases. Discov Med 2013;15(81):73–83.
15. Maheshwari R, Mack CD, Kaufman RP, et al. Severity of injury and outcomes among obese trauma patients with fractures of the femur and tibia: a crash injury research and engineering network study. J Orthop Trauma 2009;23(9):634–9.
16. Finkelstein EA, Chen H, Prabhu M, et al. The relationship between obesity and injuries among U.S. adults. Am J Health Promot 2007;21(5):460–8.
17. Takeda S, Elefteriou F, Levasseur R, et al. Leptin regulates bone formation via the sympathetic nervous system. Cell 2002;111(3):305–17.
18. Ducy P, Amling M, Takeda S, et al. Leptin inhibits bone formation through a hypothalamic relay: a central control of bone mass. Cell 2000;100(2):197–207.
19. Einhorn TA. Brain, bone, and body mass: fat is beautiful again. J Bone Joint Surg Am 2001;83-A(12):1782.
20. Haberland M, Schilling AF, Rueger JM, et al. Brain and bone: central regulation of bone mass. A new paradigm in skeletal biology. J Bone Joint Surg Am 2001;83-A(12):1871–6.
21. Sato M, Takeda N, Sarui H, et al. Association between serum leptin concentrations and bone mineral density, and biochemical markers of bone turnover in adult men. J Clin Endocrinol Metab 2001;86(11):5273–6.
22. Templeton DL, Kelly AS, Steinberger J, et al. Lower relative bone mineral content in obese adolescents: role of non-weight bearing exercise. Pediatr Exerc Sci 2010;22(4):557–68.
23. Sabharwal S, Root MZ. Impact of obesity on orthopaedics. J Bone Joint Surg Am 2012;94(11):1045–52.
24. Anakwenze O, Fokin A, Chocas M, et al. Complications in total shoulder and reverse total shoulder arthroplasty by body mass index. J Shoulder Elbow Surg 2017;26(7):1230–7.
25. Samson AJ, Mercer GE, Campbell DG. Total knee replacement in the morbidly obese: a literature review. ANZ J Surg 2010;80(9):595–9.

26. Werner BC, Burrus MT, Browne JA, et al. Supero-besity (body mass index >50 kg/m2) and complica-tions after total shoulder arthroplasty: an incremental effect of increasing body mass index. J Shoulder Elbow Surg 2015;24(12):1868–75.

27. Browne JA. CORR insights((R)): obesity epidemic: is its impact on total joint arthroplasty underesti-mated? An analysis of national trends. Clin Orthop Relat Res 2017;475(7):1807–8.

28. Collins JE, Donnell-Fink LA, Yang HY, et al. Effect of obesity on pain and functional recovery following total knee arthroplasty. J Bone Joint Surg Am 2017;99(21):1812–8.

29. Edelstein AI, Suleiman LI, Alvarez AP, et al. The interaction of obesity and metabolic syndrome in determining risk of complication following total joint arthroplasty. J Arthroplasty 2016;31(9 Suppl): 192–6.

30. Fehring TK, Odum SM, Griffin WL, et al. The obesity epidemic: its effect on total joint arthro-plasty. J Arthroplasty 2007;22(6 Suppl 2):71–6.

31. Fournier MN, Hallock J, Mihalko WM. Preoperative optimization of total joint arthroplasty surgical risk: obesity. J Arthroplasty 2016;31(8):1620–4.

32. Fu MC, D'Ambrosia C, McLawhorn AS, et al. Malnutrition increases with obesity and is a stron-ger independent risk factor for postoperative com-plications: a propensity-adjusted analysis of total hip arthroplasty patients. J Arthroplasty 2016; 31(11):2415–21.

33. George J, Klika AK, Navale SM, et al. Obesity epidemic: is its impact on total joint arthroplasty underestimated? An analysis of national trends. Clin Orthop Relat Res 2017;475(7):1798–806.

34. Hanly RJ, Marvi SK, Whitehouse SL, et al. Morbid obesity in total hip arthroplasty: redefin-ing outcomes for operative time, length of stay, and readmission. J Arthroplasty 2016;31(9): 1949–53.

35. Houdek MT, Wagner ER, Watts CD, et al. Morbid obesity: a significant risk factor for failure of two-stage revision total hip arthroplasty for infection. J Bone Joint Surg Am 2015;97(4):326–32.

36. Inacio MC, Kritz-Silverstein D, Raman R, et al. The risk of surgical site infection and re-admission in obese patients undergoing total joint replacement who lose weight before surgery and keep it off post-operatively. Bone Joint J 2014;96-B(5):629–35.

37. Kandil A, Werner BC, Gwathmey WF, et al. Obesity, morbid obesity and their related medical comor-bidities are associated with increased complica-tions and revision rates after unicompartmental knee arthroplasty. J Arthroplasty 2015;30(3):456–60.

38. Li W, Ayers DC, Lewis CG, et al. Functional gain and pain relief after total joint replacement accord-ing to obesity status. J Bone Joint Surg Am 2017; 99(14):1183–9.

39. Martin JR, Jennings JM, Dennis DA. Morbid obesity and total knee arthroplasty: a growing problem. J Am Acad Orthop Surg 2017;25(3): 188–94.

40. Murgatroyd SE, Frampton CM, Wright MS. The ef-fect of body mass index on outcome in total hip arthroplasty: early analysis from the New Zealand joint registry. J Arthroplasty 2014;29(10):1884–8.

41. Schipper ON, Denduluri SK, Zhou Y, et al. Effect of obesity on total ankle arthroplasty outcomes. Foot Ankle Int 2016;37(1):1–7.

42. Wagner ER, Houdek MT, Schleck C, et al. Increasing body mass index is associated with worse outcomes after shoulder arthroplasty. J Bone Joint Surg Am 2017;99(11):929–37.

43. Ward DT, Metz LN, Horst PK, et al. Complications of morbid obesity in total joint arthroplasty: risk stratification based on BMI. J Arthroplasty 2015; 30(9 Suppl):42–6.

44. Rasmussen JV, Olsen BS, Fevang BT, et al. A review of national shoulder and elbow joint replacement registries. J Shoulder Elbow Surg 2012;21(10): 1328–35.

45. Jo S, Morrey BF, Sanchez-Sotelo J, et al. A 40 year experience in primary elbow arthroplasty: a study of 1299 elbows. AAOS 2015 Annual Meeting. Sands Expo and Convention Center. Las Vegas (NV), March 24–28, 2015.

46. Goodnough LH, Finlay AK, Huddleston JI 3rd, et al. Obesity is independently associated with early aseptic loosening in primary total hip arthroplasty. J Arthroplasty 2017;33(3):882–6.

47. Griffin JW, Novicoff WM, Browne JA, et al. Morbid obesity in total shoulder arthroplasty: risk, out-comes, and cost analysis. J Shoulder Elbow Surg 2014;23(10):1444–8.

48. Gupta AK, Chalmers PN, Rahman Z, et al. Reverse total shoulder arthroplasty in patients of varying body mass index. J Shoulder Elbow Surg 2014; 23(1):35–42.

49. Pappou I, Virani NA, Clark R, et al. Outcomes and costs of reverse shoulder arthroplasty in the morbidly obese: a case control study. J Bone Joint Surg Am 2014;96(14):1169–76.

50. Statz JM, Wagner ER, Houdek MT, et al. Outcomes of primary reverse shoulder arthroplasty in patients with morbid obesity. J Shoulder Elbow Surg 2016; 25(7):e191–198.

51. Werner BC, Burrus MT, Begho I, et al. Early revision within 1 year after shoulder arthroplasty: patient factors and etiology. J Shoulder Elbow Surg 2015; 24(12):e323–330.

52. Werner BC, Griffin JW, Yang S, et al. Obesity is associated with increased postoperative complica-tions after operative management of proximal hu-merus fractures. J Shoulder Elbow Surg 2015; 24(4):593–600.

53. Werner BC, Rawles RB, Jobe JT, et al. Obesity is associated with increased postoperative complications after operative management of distal humerus fractures. J Shoulder Elbow Surg 2015;24(10):1602–6.

54. Griffin JW, Werner BC, Gwathmey FW, et al. Obesity is associated with increased postoperative complications after total elbow arthroplasty. J Shoulder Elbow Surg 2015;24(10):1594–601.

55. Large R, Tambe A, Cresswell T, et al. Medium-term clinical results of a linked total elbow replacement system. Bone Joint J 2014;96-B(10):1359–65.

56. Baghdadi YM, Veillette CJ, Malone AA, et al. Total elbow arthroplasty in obese patients. J Bone Joint Surg Am 2014;96(9):e70.

57. Collins JA, Beutel BG, Garofolo G, et al. Correlation of obesity with patient-reported outcomes and complications after hip arthroscopy. Arthroscopy 2015;31(1):57–62.

58. Handschin AE, Trentz OA, Hemmi S, et al. Leptin increases extracellular matrix mineralization of human osteoblasts from heterotopic ossification and normal bone. Ann Plast Surg 2007;59(3):329–33.

59. Ikeda Y, Nakajima A, Aiba A, et al. Association between serum leptin and bone metabolic markers, and the development of heterotopic ossification of the spinal ligament in female patients with ossification of the posterior longitudinal ligament. Eur Spine J 2011;20(9):1450–8.

60. Koelbl O, Seufert J, Pohl F, et al. Preoperative irradiation for prevention of heterotopic ossification following prosthetic total hip replacement results of a prospective study in 462 hips. Strahlenther Onkol 2003;179(11):767–73.

61. Mourad WF, Packianathan S, Shourbaji RA, et al. The impact of class III (morbid) obesity on heterotopic ossification outcomes. Pract Radiat Oncol 2012;2(3):e1–6.

62. Salazar D, Golz A, Israel H, et al. Heterotopic ossification of the elbow treated with surgical resection: risk factors, bony ankylosis, and complications. Clin Orthop Relat Res 2014;472(7):2269–75.

63. Yushuva A, Nagda P, Suzuki K, et al. Heterotopic mesenteric ossification following gastric bypass surgery: case series and review of literature. Obes Surg 2010;20(9):1312–5.

64. Plaschke HC, Thillemann TM, Brorson S, et al. Implant survival after total elbow arthroplasty: a retrospective study of 324 procedures performed from 1980 to 2008. J Shoulder Elbow Surg 2014; 23:829–36.

65. Kraay MJ, Figgie MP, Inglis AE, et al. Primary semiconstrained total elbow arthroplasty. Survival analysis of 113 consecutive cases. J Bone Joint Surg Br 1994;76:636–40.

66. Sanchez-Sotelo J. Total elbow arthroplasty. Open Orthop J 2011;5:115–23.

Foot and Ankle

Foot and Ankle

Obesity in Elective Foot and Ankle Surgery

Matthew Stewart, MD

KEYWORDS

- Obesity • Elective surgery • Foot and ankle surgery • Total ankle replacements
- Body mass index • Forefoot surgery • Ankle arthroscopy

KEY POINTS

- The prevalence of obesity is increasing at a staggering rate. Obesity is related to many comorbidities, including heart disease, diabetes, metabolic syndrome, and musculoskeletal disorders. Caring for obese patients is proving to be a significant financial burden to our health care dollars.
- Obese patients have been found to have higher rates of foot and ankle pain, likely because of a complex interplay between alterations in gait, increased biomechanical loads, and metabolic effects of excess adipose tissue.
- There is conflicting evidence as to whether obese patients are at increased risk of complications following total ankle replacements, ankle arthroscopy, flatfoot reconstruction, and forefoot surgery.
- It is important to counsel obese patients about weight loss and other modifiable comorbid conditions before elective surgical intervention.

INTRODUCTION

The waistlines of Americans are expanding at an alarming rate. By now it is a well-known fact that we are in the midst of an obesity epidemic. Epidemic is a powerful word, but it perfectly encapsulates the extensiveness of the problem. Obesity has wide-ranging effects with serious health and economic consequences. As society has become more technologically advanced, we have begun to live more sedentary lifestyles. We are at a point now where much of our needs are met with the touch of a button. Shopping, learning, working, entertainment, and communication can be addressed in the seated position with our mobile or laptop devices. Multiple studies highlight that children and adolescents are becoming increasingly less active, with most not participating in the recommended 1 hour of daily physical activity.[1] It only makes sense that we would see these rising rates of obesity. In 1960, 16% of women and 12% of men were considered obese.[2] By 2008, the vast majority, more than 68% of US adults were overweight and 35% of women and 32% of men were considered obese.[3] That was 10 years ago, so rest assured the rates are even higher at this point because the trend is only increasing. In fact, if the present trend continues at this rate, by 2030, 86% of adults will be overweight and more than 50% will be obese.[4] These staggering numbers are a growing drain to our health care dollars as well. Obesity carries with it a significant burden of disease. Diabetes, high blood pressure, coronary artery disease, stroke, high cholesterol, asthma, arthritis, and overall poor health status are associated with being overweight.[5,6] Quality-adjusted life-years (QALYs) is used as a generic measurement tool for morbidity and mortality associated with a disease process. It is used to assess different diseases and compare them so that the degree to which they affect overall health can be quantified. From 1993 to 2008, the average QALYs

Disclosure Statement: The author has no conflicts of interest or disclosures.
The Hughston Clinic, 6262 Veterans Parkway, Columbus, GA 31908, USA
E-mail address: mgstewart@hughston.com

Orthop Clin N Am 49 (2018) 371–379
https://doi.org/10.1016/j.ocl.2018.02.011
0030-5898/18/© 2018 Elsevier Inc. All rights reserved.

loss increased 127% for obesity, making it an even greater contributor to morbidity than smoking.[7,8] We are now spending in excess of 100 billion dollars each year on health care resources that are attributed to obesity.[6] That number is expected to double every decade, and by 2030, 1 in every 6 health care dollar has been projected toward an obesity-related health complication.[4]

Presently, the vast majority of obesity-related orthopedic literature has been derived from hip and knee arthroplasty studies. Within total joint arthroplasty, it has been well established that obesity increases perioperative complications and leads to higher rates of revisions and reoperations.[9–17] It has only been over the last few years that publications have highlighted the effects of obesity on foot and ankle surgery. The purpose of this article is to provide a comprehensive review of the literature as it pertains to obesity within foot and ankle surgery, with hopes of improving surgeon decision making, mitigating risk, and providing better outcomes for patients. A better understanding of the effects of obesity also allows for improved prognostic performance, which plays a substantial role in patient education, especially when counseling about potential surgical risks and benefits. Increased patient awareness should only aid the patient and surgeon if complications do arise. If realistic expectations have been set beforehand, then each side should be better equipped to deal with difficulties that will invariably arise. Areas of concern for obese patients undergoing foot and ankle surgery may also be identified and it may be determined if there are specific pathologic conditions where the current literature is deficient, with the goal of establishing areas of future research.

DEFINING OBESITY

Obesity has been defined by the World Health Organization as a body mass index (BMI) greater than 30. BMI is a calculation based on a person's weight and height. This scale is used as a screening tool given its ease of collection and cost-effectiveness. It is also the metric used by most research studies when discussing obesity, making it very easy for comparative data analysis. The use of BMI has been criticized though because it may falsely identify muscular individuals as obese, given that it cannot distinguish the weight of muscle versus that of fat. It also does not take into account the distribution of adipose tissue. Waist circumference and measurement of the percentage of body fat have also been used to define obesity but to a lesser extent.

BIOMECHANICAL AND METABOLIC EFFECT OF OBESITY

Both biomechanical and metabolic mechanisms have been hypothesized to contribute to the high rates of orthopedic pathologic condition in obese patients. The foot and ankle provide the base of support during standing and walking, so intuitively, it makes sense from a biomechanical standpoint that obesity would have a significant effect. Traditional views were that excess weight places additional stress across bones and soft tissues and will eventually lead to "wear and tear," putting these patients at increased risk for arthritis, tendonitis, and bursitis. These injuries are often colloquially termed "overuse injuries," and it seems logical to assume that obese patients would suffer more frequently from these conditions. Frey and Zamora[18] surveyed 1411 subjects and found that patients with a BMI greater than 25 were more likely to have tendinitis within the foot and ankle compared with the control group (BMI <25). Riddle and colleagues[19] found that patients with BMI greater than 30 were at increased risk of developing plantar fasciitis. To make matters worse, Weil[20] found that patients with a higher BMI had less success with typical conservative treatments for Achilles tendinopathy, plantar fasciitis, and adult-onset posterior tibial tendon dysfunction. These treatment failures may be the result of decreased healing potential, as related to metabolic factors discussed later, or difficultly with common conservative treatment methods, such as body habitus, limiting the effectiveness of brace-wear or therapeutic exercises.

Obese patients also have more foot and ankle pain in general compared with normal weight subjects.[21–23] Mickle and Steele[21] looked at more than 300 subjects divided into 3 groups based on weight: normal, overweight, and obese. Foot pain was present in 40% of the obese compared with 23% of the overweight and 11% of the normal weight. They hypothesized these findings were secondary to changes in the normal biomechanics of the foot and ankle during standing and walking. At baseline, obese subjects have significant reductions in gait speed, resulting in increased total contact time with the ground during stance phase and increased peak pressure across the midfoot. Excessive biomechanical loading with a foot that is in contact with the ground longer leads to these painful foot and ankle conditions, causing alterations in the gait cycle and potential changes to the shape of the foot. Obese children and adults were found to have flatter, wider feet with significantly larger contact areas that generated larger forces across the plantar surface of their total foot: heel, midfoot, and forefoot.[24,25] It is theorized that this increased pressure exposes the plantar surface to increased stress and in turn makes the bones and soft tissues vulnerable to further damage.[24] This can perpetuate a vicious cycle in attempts to avoid pain, with further alterations in gait that lead to changes in force distribution across the foot and contribute to worsening symptoms.

Many additional observational studies also support the fact that obese patients suffer from chronic foot and ankle pain and overuse injuries more frequently.[26–30] Unfortunately, there is a paucity of scientific foot and ankle literature to support the biomechanical theory in isolation. Although limited, there are a few studies examining the biomechanical interaction between excessive joint loading and the development of knee osteoarthritis. There seems to be interplay between muscle fatigue and biomechanical changes seen at the knee joint. Obese patients have been shown to have reductions in quadriceps strength earlier with walking, leading to faster fatigue, decreased shock attenuation, and increased loading rate across the joint.[31,32] Experimental studies have also shown that specific loading conditions can lead to changes at the molecular level on chondrocytes. Chondrocytes demonstrate mechanoreceptors that are sensitive to pressure. Their response to increased loads may lead to increased expression of metalloproteases and cytokines that can trigger matrix synthesis inhibition and cartilage degeneration. Consequently, obesity could potentiate arthritic changes at the cellular level through a complex biomechanical/metabolic pathway.[33,34]

The metabolic component alone is a bit more complicated. Adipose tissue can be thought of as an endocrine organ in itself, so excess fat accumulation results in a more powerful organ with metabolic implications. Adipose tissue secretes numerous cytokines collectively known as adipokines. Many of these adipokines are of an inflammatory nature and have a negative effect on metabolism. It is theorized that they produce a state of constant, low grade inflammation, which has been proposed as the underlying cause of metabolic syndrome. Metabolic syndrome represents an association between central obesity with the presence of elevated cardiovascular risk factors, such as hypertension,

insulin resistance, and atherogenic dyslipidemia. This proinflammatory environment also has deleterious effects on the musculoskeletal system, and some have proposed adding osteoarthritis to this syndrome, because it shares many common mediators and pathways as the cardiovascular risk factors.[35,36] Many of these inflammatory cytokines have the potential to weaken bones, affect bony and soft tissue healing, and contribute to increased complications seen within obese populations, such as infection or deep vein thrombosis. Cohen and colleagues[37] showed that excess abdominal fat was associated with lower bone formation and inferior bone quality. In his healthy premenopausal subjects, trunk fat was associated with greater cortical porosity, decreased stiffness, and less trabecular bone volume. Cao[38] suggests that increased levels of circulating inflammatory cytokines may promote increased bone resorption through activation of the RANK/RANK ligand system of osteoclastic activity. Both of these views dispute traditional views that obesity should be protective of bone health given the well-established effect that excessive mechanical loading should increase bone formation, that is, Wolff's law. There are other mediators at play as well. Both calcium and vitamin D pathways are affected by obesity. High-fat diets will decrease the amount of calcium absorbed in the intestines, thus decreasing availability for bone formation. Goldner and colleagues[39] found that 90% of patients were vitamin D deficient before undergoing bariatric surgery for weight loss. There has always been a concern that these patients would be at risk for vitamin deficiency after surgery given the changes in stomach and intestinal absorption that occur postoperatively. The results of Coupaye and colleagues[40] dispute this. Coupaye and colleagues[40] evaluated 202 obese patients and found that 80% were vitamin D deficient before their bariatric surgery. The serum vitamin D level increased from an average of 13.4 preoperatively to 22.8 postoperatively, and the percentage of vitamin D–deficient patients reduced to 44%. They concluded that excessive weight was the reason for their low vitamin D levels and that weight loss had a greater influence on vitamin D levels rather than malabsorption induced by gastric bypass.

The available evidence is clear that obesity results in an increased prevalence of numerous orthopedic conditions, although the mechanisms are still not completely understood. Although there seems to be contributions from both a biomechanical standpoint and systemic inflammation, the exact interplay between the 2 is still not completely understood. Further basic science research is necessary to understand, treat, and potentially prevent the damaging effects of obesity on the musculoskeletal system.

OBESITY-RELATED SURGICAL ISSUES

Obesity can present unique challenges for both the surgeon and the patient. Patients with excess adipose tissue can experience more difficult surgeries because visualization may be compromised, larger incisions are often required, and the operating times are often longer when compared with nonobese patients. In addition, there is theoretic evidence to suggest that obese patients may have compromised wound healing. In this area, as with most metabolic, obesity-related issues, the exact mechanism is complex, multifactorial, and more than likely, not completely understood. Wound healing may be influenced by the deleterious effect of the inflammatory adipokines secreted excessively in obese patients. It has also been hypothesized that relative hypoperfusion exists locally at the wound caused by increased adipose tissue and wound tension. This hypoperfusion can lead to decreased delivery of antibiotics and reduced availability of oxygen at the surgical incision.[41–43] Combine this with confounding comorbidities, such as diabetes and peripheral vascular disease, the aforementioned longer operating times, and larger incisions, and a complex relationship exists of risk factors that have the potential to increase postoperative complications. These risks can result in longer hospital stays and increased rates of hospital discharge to skilled nursing facilities, all of which serve to increase health care dollars.

After foot and ankle surgery, patients are commonly placed in a cast or splint and instructed to maintain non-weight-bearing on the operative extremity while bones and soft tissues are allowed to heal. This immobilization creates difficulties even for the healthiest of patients, because of risk of falls or potential risk of deep vein thrombosis that accompanies immobility. Ambulation while non-weight-bearing on 1 extremity may be even more difficult in obese patients, because of balance issues or just overall difficultly using crutches or a walker because of their size. This may potentially lead to noncompliance of the weight-bearing restriction. After surgery, particularly fracture fixation or bony fusion, noncompliance with weight-bearing may compromise the internal fixation and load to micromotion across the bony interface and potential for nonunion and/or hardware

failure. This would constitute a major complication, likely requiring revision surgery with all the additional risk that accompanies returning to the operating room.

These issues need to be addressed with patients and their family before surgery. They need to be aware of potential risks as well as the difficulty they may encounter even with routine postoperative care. There may be potential social or medical barriers that can be addressed on the front end, such as a discussing weight loss or addressing comorbidities with the patient's primary care physicians to optimize their medical health. A referral to a physical therapist preoperatively for "pretherapy" has been proven beneficial and cost-effective. Just 1 or 2 visits for training on gait-assistance devices and planning strategies for recovery with family members has helped reduce postoperative care.[44] Surgical decision making before elective foot and ankle surgery is a time not only to explain the risk and benefits of a procedure but also when realistic expectations should be addressed. This honest communication should not only improve the patient-surgeon interaction but also allow for more informed decision making.

TOTAL ANKLE REPLACEMENT

With the advent of third-generation implants during the last decade, total ankle replacement has been accepted as a reliable treatment option for end-stage arthritis. One of the biggest concerns initially had been durability, because initial designs had failed early and often because of loosening and subsidence of the components. The recent literature has shown these newer, more anatomically designed implants to be quite durable with survivorship consistently greater than 90% at 5 to 10 years postoperatively.[45–47] Although with this historical perspective, it begs the question as to whether obese patients could expect the same success with the inevitable increased loads seen across their prosthesis. The literature from hip and knee arthroplasty suggests that obese patients are more likely to require revision surgery and have early postoperative complications, such as infection and deep vein thrombosis.[9–11,15,16,48,49] Also, although these patients have high satisfaction ratings and significant improvements in their functional outcomes, their results are lower overall than their normal weight counterparts.[11,50,51] Up to this point, there are only a few publications specifically looking at obesity's effects on total ankle arthroplasty. Gross and colleagues[52] retrospectively looked at 455 primary total ankles with a minimum of 2-year follow-up. Patients were categorized into 3 groups based on BMI (<30, 30–35, and >35). Their results showed that although obese patients did experience significant pain and functional improvements, their functional outcome scores were significantly lower than the control group. They did not find higher complications, revisions, or infection rates. Bouchard and colleagues[53] compared 39 obese patients with 48 nonobese patients and also found no difference in the proportion of complications or revisions. Also, although the obese group had worse disability and function before surgery, they still similarly and significantly improved their pain and disability scores. Barg and colleagues[54] looked specifically at component stability and found no association between an increased BMI and increased radiographic evidence of loosening at an average of 5.5-year follow-up.

There are a few studies the results of which contradict the notion that obese patients will do equally as well after total ankle replacement. Schipper and colleagues[55] reported 97 total ankle replacements and found that the obese group had a significantly higher probability toward failure and revision surgery compared with the nonobese group. Interestingly, when the obese group was stratified by cause, the obese patients with osteoarthritis had a higher failure rate at 5 years compared with obese patients with posttraumatic or inflammatory arthritis. It should be noted that this study has an overall failure rate, for both obese and nonobese, that is significantly higher than the vast majority of reported total ankle outcomes. The author contributes this to the use of a second-generation implant that is no longer available for use in the United States. Also, their criterion for failure includes exchange of the polyethylene component, whereas most comparative studies include this in reoperation rate but not component failure. In another study that examined a database of greater than 23,000 patients treated for end-stage ankle arthritis, they found that obese patients with total ankle replacement had significantly more major and minor complications at 90 days, including infection and venous thromboembolism. They also showed an increased incidence of revision surgery in the obese group.[56]

To date, there is no study that directly links obesity with altered implant loading that leads to subsidence or failure of the prosthesis. One radiostereometric study did demonstrate that implants will subside over time under load and that the area of subsidence correlates with the direction of primary loading.[57] Although this study was not designed to look at the effects of obesity on implant loading, it does seem logical to infer that patients with increased weight would have higher joint reaction forces across the ankle and potentially cause early migration and failure.

ANKLE ARTHROSCOPY

Ankle arthroscopy is a useful tool in the armamentarium of any foot and ankle surgeon. It is commonly used for treatment of ankle impingement, talus osteochondral lesions (OCLs), removal of loose bodies, and minimally invasive ankle fusions. Anterolateral ankle impingement occurs because of hypertrophy of the distal aspects of the anterior tibiofibular ligament and can arise as a chronic manifestation of an ankle sprain. Approximately 1% to 2% of ankle inversion injuries can require arthroscopic treatment of impingement lesions.[58] Mardani-Kivi and colleagues[58] looked at the effect of obesity on the success of arthroscopic treatment of these impingement lesions. Twenty-six obese patients (BMI >30) and 10 nonobese patients were examined at 6 and 12 months following surgery using the American Orthopaedic Foot and Ankle Society (AOFAS) scores. At 1-year follow-up, the presence of obesity had no effect on the effectiveness of treatment, but obese patients were found to have a significantly higher prevalence of associated chondral lesions at the time of surgery (58% vs 30%). Although outcomes were not affected by this in the short term, there is potential that these chondral lesions could lead to higher morbidity at longer-term follow-up.

Talus OCLs can be challenging problems for orthopedic surgeons. A variety of potential reasons have been cited for the development of OCLs, including congenital and traumatic causes. Although guidelines are in place to help guide a surgeon's decision to treat these surgically, there is still no general consensus on what type of surgical treatment is best. Marrow stimulation techniques, osteochondral transplant, autologous chondrocyte implantation, and bulk allograft have all been used with varying degrees of success. Usuelli and colleagues[59] assessed their results of autologous matrix-induced chondrogenesis for the treatment of talar OCLs in 2 groups of patients that were divided based on weight (BMI <25 or >25). They found that although overweight patients were more likely to have larger lesions based on preoperative MRIs, this did not translate into worse functional outcomes at 24-month follow-up, because both groups showed similar clinical improvements. In contrast with those results, Chuckpaiwong and colleagues[60] found that higher BMI was a significant predictor of a negative outcome in their analysis of 105 patients who underwent microfracture for their talus OCL. At this point, the impact of weight on the treatment of OCLs is still unknown. The few studies published have conflicting evidence and different treatment protocols. As with most obesity-related foot and ankle studies, more patients and longer follow-up are necessary to understand the true relationship.

FLATFOOT

Epidemiologic studies suggest that obese individuals are more likely to develop posterior tibial tendon dysfunction, but to date there are very little clinical data to guide decision making for obese patients with a flexible deformity.[28,29] The gold standard for a flexible pes planovalgus deformity has been reconstruction through osteotomies and tendon transfers to realign the foot and restore the arch. The concern is that obese patients will cause premature reoccurrence of the deformity because reconstruction may not be powerful enough to withstand their excessive biomechanical loads. The alternative is realignment by arthrodesis of the hindfoot and transverse tarsal joints. Obviously though, avoidance of an unnecessary fusion is attractive to the patient and physician because joint motion would be preserved, function would be improved, and secondary adjacent joint arthritis that can occur after arthrodesis would be prevented. However, for argument's sake, suppose a reconstruction was performed and prematurely failed (ie, reoccurrence of the deformity, failure to correct the deformity, or continued pain). This failure would be a significant burden to the patient. The patient would now require a second major operation on the foot and ankle with all the associated consequences and risks of surgery. A second surgery likely means an additional 6 to 12 weeks of non-weight-bearing and immobilization, potentially more time lost from work, additional physical therapy, and the inconvenience of returning for multiple postoperative visits. For these reasons, understanding what prognostic factors may lead to an unsuccessful reconstruction would be highly beneficial. Specifically, is there a certain BMI cutoff for obese patients that would lead to more reliable results with an initial arthrodesis rather than a flexible flatfoot reconstruction?

Soukup and colleagues[61] reported their clinical and radiographic outcomes following reconstruction of stage II adult acquired flatfoot deformity. They had 44 normal weight patients, 39 overweight patients, and 44 obese patients with a mean follow-up of 2.9 years. They concluded that obese patients had significantly worse symptoms, pain, and overall health preoperatively, but short-term clinical and radiographic outcomes were similar across all patient groups. Also, although the overall complications were higher with an increased BMI, these results did not reach significance. This study would suggest that obese patients are still a candidate for reconstruction with comparable results in the short term, but more patients and longer follow-up are necessary to determine if these results are durable over time under increased loads.

FOREFOOT SURGERY

Hallux valgus is one of the most common elective procedures within the foot and ankle area. The effect of obesity has been looked at in terms of surgical correction as well as the risk of developing this deformity. Chen and colleagues[62] investigated the effect of obesity on functional outcomes and recurrence rate following hallux valgus surgery. They prospectively followed 452 surgical patients and categorized them into 2 groups based on BMI greater than or less than 30. Obese patients were found to have comparable outcomes scores on the Visual Analogue Scale, AOFAS Hallux Metatarsophalangeal-Interphalangeal scale, physical and mental component scores, as well as rates of surgical sites infection, although the obese group was found to have a significantly higher percentage of reoperations (14% vs 2%), primarily because of hardware irritation and reoccurrence of their bunion deformity. The investigators postulated this was due to physical problems caused by obesity that can lead to technical difficulties with hardware insertion and surgical correction. They also were concerned that the effect of obesity on bony healing could have led to higher rates of recurrence and nonunion. Milczarek and colleagues[63] reported on 132 hallux valgus patients treated with a scarf osteotomy. They found that obese patients had similar radiographic results and no significant differences in pain, functional outcomes, or satisfaction ratings. Stewart and colleagues[41] looked at the effect of obesity on all of their elective forefoot surgery patients. They retrospectively reviewed 633 patients and found similar complication rates between the obese (10%) and nonobese (9%) cohorts. They did find that diabetics were significantly more likely to develop a surgical site infection, regardless of weight, and there was an overall trend toward increased complications in the diabetics as well.

Elective forefoot surgery may be less susceptible to obesity, in that surgeries are often shorter and are performed under regional anesthesia, and patients are often allowed to weight-bear, at least partially, after surgery. This means easier recoveries, alleviating many of the concerns that accompany non-weight-bearing and the potential risks of decreased immobilization. The forefoot also has limited subcutaneous fat comparatively, which may be protective against some of the factors that lead to wound complications. Smaller, less extensive dissections mean less risk of developing hematomas, seromas, or wound dehiscence.

SUMMARY

When trying to decide whether to pursue elective surgery, the major question left for surgeons and their patients is, "Are the risks worth the rewards?" This question is particularly pertinent when dealing with obesity because it is one of the few modifiable risk factors that can help push the scale in the direction of a favorable outcome. It used to be that the surgeon and patient could have a long discussion detailing the facts of surgery and the additional risk that may come with a particular comorbidity, and if they both decided that those risks were acceptable, then they could proceed with surgery. Now, a time has come whereby health care policy is starting to play a role in these types of decisions. Government legislation and hospital regulations have begun to limit access to certain surgeries for obese patients based on arbitrary BMI thresholds. The financial risk of a complication outweighs the reward. Physicians may also have less incentive to proceed with surgery on at-risk patients. Because reimbursement methods become linked to surgical outcomes, there is less financial incentive to operate on patients with significant comorbidities because of the risk of a complication. Reimbursement has been discussed a great deal in terms of the new "bundled" payments for joint arthroplasty. These surgeries have a set price for the hospital and the surgeon, so if a complication causes the spending to exceed the predetermined price, the hospital and surgeon would be required to cover the difference. These potential patients have been referred to as the "bundle breakers,"

and their potential has serious ramifications as to the way health care decisions will be made.

There is still much to learn about the effect obesity has on foot and ankle surgery. At this point, there are only a few studies looking at just a handful of foot and ankle pathologic conditions and types of surgeries. Most of these studies, unfortunately, contain only a small number of patients stratified into dichotomous groups of obese (BMI >30) and nonobese (BMI <30). This can create difficulties determining true differences in complications and outcomes because the studies are underpowered and oversimplified. In addition, most studies do not subclassify obese patients by their associated comorbidities. Many of these comorbidities, such as diabetes and peripheral vascular disease, may be the true culprit that leads to increased complications or poor outcomes. Often, the results of these studies provide contradictory evidence or lead to more questions. The answers will only be determined with continued research that has additional patients, longer follow-ups, and more specific obesity-related questions. What is known is that obesity is a growing problem that each surgeon will frequently encounter in his or her practice. Obesity has serious health consequences that can compromise overall health as well as musculoskeletal function. The orthopedic foot and ankle surgeon has a responsibility not only to address the patients' orthopedic complaints but also to help guide them in a way that promotes a more healthy and active lifestyle.

REFERENCES

1. Roman B, Serra-Majem L, Ribas-Barba L, et al. How many children and adolescents in Spain comply with the recommendations on physical activity? J Sports Med Phys Fitness 2008;48(3):380–7.
2. Ogden CL, Carroll MD, Kit BK, et al. Prevalence of obesity in the United States, 2009-2010. NCHS Data Brief 2012;82:1–8.
3. Flegal KM, Carroll MD, Ogden CL, et al. Prevalence and trends in obesity among US adults, 1999-2008. JAMA 2010;303(3):235–41.
4. Wang Y, Beydoun MA, Liang L, et al. Will all Americans become overweight or obese? Estimating the progression and cost of the US obesity epidemic. Obesity (Silver Spring) 2008;16(10):2323–30.
5. Mokdad AH, Ford ES, Bowman BA, et al. Prevalence of obesity, diabetes, and obesity-related health risk factors, 2001. JAMA 2003;289(1):76–9.
6. Thompson D, Edelsberg J, Colditz GA, et al. Lifetime health and economic consequences of obesity. Arch Intern Med 1999;159(18):2177–83.

7. Jia H, Lubetkin EI. Obesity-related quality-adjusted life years lost in the U.S. from 1993 to 2008. Am J Prev Med 2010;39(3):220–7.

8. Jia H, Lubetkin EI. Trends in quality-adjusted life-years lost contributed by smoking and obesity. Am J Prev Med 2010;38(2):138–44.

9. Haverkamp D, Klinkenbijl MN, Somford MP, et al. Obesity in total hip arthroplasty–does it really matter? A meta-analysis. Acta Orthop 2011;82(4):417–22.

10. Kerkhoffs GM, Servien E, Dunn W, et al. The influence of obesity on the complication rate and outcome of total knee arthroplasty: a meta-analysis and systematic literature review. J Bone Joint Surg Am 2012;94(20):1839–44.

11. Baker P, Petheram T, Jameson S, et al. The association between body mass index and the outcomes of total knee arthroplasty. J Bone Joint Surg Am 2012;94(16):1501–8.

12. Wagner ER, Houdek MT, Schleck C, et al. Increasing body mass index is associated with worse outcomes after shoulder arthroplasty. J Bone Joint Surg Am 2017;99(11):929–37.

13. Workgroup of the American Association of Hip and Knee Surgeons Evidence Based Committee. Obesity and total joint arthroplasty: a literature based review. J Arthroplasty 2013;28(5):714–21.

14. Schwarzkopf R, Thompson SL, Adwar SJ, et al. Postoperative complication rates in the "super-obese" hip and knee arthroplasty population. J Arthroplasty 2012;27(3):397–401.

15. Jamsen E, Nevalainen P, Eskelinen A, et al. Obesity, diabetes, and preoperative hyperglycemia as predictors of periprosthetic joint infection: a single-center analysis of 7181 primary hip and knee replacements for osteoarthritis. J Bone Joint Surg Am 2012;94(14):e101.

16. Namba RS, Inacio MC, Paxton EW. Risk factors associated with surgical site infection in 30,491 primary total hip replacements. J Bone Joint Surg Br 2012;94(10):1330–8.

17. Kamath AF, McAuliffe CL, Baldwin KD, et al. Unplanned admission to the intensive care unit after total hip arthroplasty. J Arthroplasty 2012;27(6):1027–32.e1-2.

18. Frey C, Zamora J. The effects of obesity on orthopaedic foot and ankle pathology. Foot Ankle Int 2007;28(9):996–9.

19. Riddle DL, Pulisic M, Pidcoe P, et al. Risk factors for plantar fasciitis: a matched case-control study. J Bone Joint Surg Am 2003;85-A(5):872–7.

20. Weil L Jr. Obesity, feet, and the impact on health care. Foot Ankle Spec 2012;5(3):148–9.

21. Mickle KJ, Steele JR. Obese older adults suffer foot pain and foot-related functional limitation. Gait Posture 2015;42(4):442–7.

22. Tanamas SK, Wluka AE, Berry P, et al. Relationship between obesity and foot pain and its association with fat mass, fat distribution, and muscle mass. Arthritis Care Res (Hoboken) 2012;64(2):262–8.

23. Perruccio AV, Gandhi R, Lau JT, et al. Cross-sectional contrast between individuals with foot/ankle vs knee osteoarthritis for obesity and low education on health-related quality of life. Foot Ankle Int 2016;37(1):24–32.

24. Mickle KJ, Steele JR, Munro BJ. Does excess mass affect plantar pressure in young children? Int J Pediatr Obes 2006;1(3):183–8.

25. Dowling AM, Steele JR, Baur LA. Does obesity influence foot structure and plantar pressure patterns in prepubescent children? Int J Obes Relat Metab Disord 2001;25(6):845–52.

26. Scott RT, Hyer CF, Granata A. The correlation of Achilles tendinopathy and body mass index. Foot Ankle Spec 2013;6(4):283–5.

27. Klein EE, Weil L Jr, Weil LS Sr, et al. Body mass index and Achilles tendonitis: a 10-year retrospective analysis. Foot Ankle Spec 2013;6(4):276–82.

28. Holmes GB Jr, Mann RA. Possible epidemiological factors associated with rupture of the posterior tibial tendon. Foot Ankle 1992;13(2):70–9.

29. Fuhrmann RA, Trommer T, Venbrocks RA. The acquired buckling-flatfoot. A foot deformity due to obesity? Orthopade 2005;34(7):682–9.

30. Sullivan J, Burns J, Adams R, et al. Musculoskeletal and activity-related factors associated with plantar heel pain. Foot Ankle Int 2015;36(1):37–45.

31. Syed IY, Davis BL. Obesity and osteoarthritis of the knee: hypotheses concerning the relationship between ground reaction forces and quadriceps fatigue in long-duration walking. Med Hypotheses 2000;54(2):182–5.

32. Koonce RC, Bravman JT. Obesity and osteoarthritis: more than just wear and tear. J Am Acad Orthop Surg 2013;21(3):161–9.

33. Pottie P, Presle N, Terlain B, et al. Obesity and osteoarthritis: more complex than predicted! Ann Rheum Dis 2006;65(11):1403–5.

34. Guilak F, Fermor B, Keefe FJ, et al. The role of biomechanics and inflammation in cartilage injury and repair. Clin Orthop Relat Res 2004;(423):17–26.

35. Katz JD, Agrawal S, Velasquez M. Getting to the heart of the matter: osteoarthritis takes its place as part of the metabolic syndrome. Curr Opin Rheumatol 2010;22(5):512–9.

36. Yoshimura N, Muraki S, Oka H, et al. Association of knee osteoarthritis with the accumulation of metabolic risk factors such as overweight, hypertension, dyslipidemia, and impaired glucose tolerance in Japanese men and women: the ROAD study. J Rheumatol 2011;38(5):921–30.

37. Cohen A, Dempster DW, Recker RR, et al. Abdominal fat is associated with lower bone formation and inferior bone quality in healthy premenopausal

women: a transiliac bone biopsy study. J Clin Endocrinol Metab 2013;98(6):2562–72.

38. Cao JJ. Effects of obesity on bone metabolism. J Orthop Surg Res 2011;6:30.

39. Goldner WS, Stoner JA, Thompson J, et al. Prevalence of vitamin D insufficiency and deficiency in morbidly obese patients: a comparison with non-obese controls. Obes Surg 2008;18(2):145–50.

40. Coupaye M, Breuil MC, Riviere P, et al. Serum vitamin D increases with weight loss in obese subjects 6 months after Roux-en-Y gastric bypass. Obes Surg 2013;23(4):486–93.

41. Stewart MS, Bettin CC, Ramsey MT, et al. Effect of obesity on outcomes of forefoot surgery. Foot Ankle Int 2016;37(5):483–7.

42. Anaya DA, Dellinger EP. The obese surgical patient: a susceptible host for infection. Surg Infect (Larchmt) 2006;7(5):473–80.

43. Guo S, Dipietro LA. Factors affecting wound healing. J Dent Res 2010;89(3):219–29.

44. Snow R, Granata J, Ruhil AV, et al. Associations between preoperative physical therapy and post-acute care utilization patterns and cost in total joint replacement. J Bone Joint Surg Am 2014;96(19):e165.

45. Stewart MG, Green CL, Adams SB Jr, et al. Midterm results of the salto talaris total ankle arthroplasty. Foot Ankle Int 2017;38(11):1215–21.

46. Hofmann KJ, Shabin ZM, Ferkel E, et al. Salto talaris total ankle arthroplasty: clinical results at a mean of 5.2 years in 78 patients treated by a single surgeon. J Bone Joint Surg Am 2016;98(24):2036–46.

47. Mann JA, Mann RA, Horton E. STAR ankle: long-term results. Foot Ankle Int 2011;32(5):S473–84.

48. Chee YH, Teoh KH, Sabnis BM, et al. Total hip replacement in morbidly obese patients with osteoarthritis: results of a prospectively matched study. J Bone Joint Surg Br 2010;92(8):1066–71.

49. Spicer DD, Pomeroy DL, Badenhausen WE, et al. Body mass index as a predictor of outcome in total knee replacement. Int Orthop 2001;25(4):246–9.

50. Collins RA, Walmsley PJ, Amin AK, et al. Does obesity influence clinical outcome at nine years following total knee replacement? J Bone Joint Surg Br 2012;94(10):1351–5.

51. Stickles B, Phillips L, Brox WT, et al. Defining the relationship between obesity and total joint arthroplasty. Obes Res 2001;9(3):219–23.

52. Gross CE, Lampley A, Green CL, et al. The effect of obesity on functional outcomes and complications in total ankle arthroplasty. Foot Ankle Int 2016;37(2):137–41.

53. Bouchard M, Amin A, Pinsker E, et al. The impact of obesity on the outcome of total ankle replacement. J Bone Joint Surg Am 2015;97(11):904–10.

54. Barg A, Knupp M, Anderson AE, et al. Total ankle replacement in obese patients: component stability, weight change, and functional outcome in 118 consecutive patients. Foot Ankle Int 2011;32(10):925–32.

55. Schipper ON, Denduluri SK, Zhou Y, et al. Effect of obesity on total ankle arthroplasty outcomes. Foot Ankle Int 2016;37(1):1–7.

56. Werner BC, Burrus MT, Looney AM, et al. Obesity is associated with increased complications after operative management of end-stage ankle arthritis. Foot Ankle Int 2015;36(8):863–70.

57. Dunbar MJ, Fong JW, Wilson DA, et al. Longitudinal migration and inducible displacement of the mobility total ankle system. Acta Orthop 2012;83(4):394–400.

58. Mardani-Kivi M, Mirbolook A, Karimi Mobarakeh M, et al. Effect of obesity on arthroscopic treatment of anterolateral impingement syndrome of the ankle. J Foot Ankle Surg 2015;54(1):13–6.

59. Usuelli FG, Maccario C, Ursino C, et al. The impact of weight on arthroscopic osteochondral talar reconstruction. Foot Ankle Int 2017;38(6):612–20.

60. Chuckpaiwong B, Berkson EM, Theodore GH. Microfracture for osteochondral lesions of the ankle: outcome analysis and outcome predictors of 105 cases. Arthroscopy 2008;24(1):106–12.

61. Soukup DS, MacMahon A, Burket JC, et al. Effect of obesity on clinical and radiographic outcomes following reconstruction of stage II adult acquired flatfoot deformity. Foot Ankle Int 2016;37(3):245–54.

62. Chen JY, Lee MJ, Rikhraj K, et al. Effect of obesity on outcome of hallux valgus surgery. Foot Ankle Int 2015;36(9):1078–83.

63. Milczarek MA, Milczarek JJ, Tomasik B, et al. Being overweight has limited effect on SCARF osteotomy outcome for hallux valgus correction. Int Orthop 2017;41(4):765–72.

Foot and Ankle Surgery in the Diabetic Population

Aaron J. Guyer, MD[a,b,c,d],*

KEYWORDS

• Diabetes • Surgery • Foot • Ankle • Orthopedic

KEY POINTS

- Foot and ankle surgery in the diabetic population has a unique set of challenges that should be considered.
- Satisfactory outcomes are possible when a surgeon recognizes these unique characteristics of diabetic patients.
- Additional surgical principles need to be applied in treating these patients.

INTRODUCTION

The incidence of obesity has been increasing worldwide over the past 3 decades. With this growth, the number of patients diagnosed with type 2 diabetes mellitus has also increased dramatically over this same period. The World Health Organization reports an estimated 422 million adults were living with diabetes in 2014, compared with 108 million in 1980. The global prevalence (age-standardized) of diabetes has nearly doubled since 1980, rising from 4.7% to 8.5% in the adult population. This reflects an increase in associated risk factors, such as being overweight or obese, and obesity is the strongest risk factor for type 2 diabetes.[1] Coincident with this surge in the number of patients who have diabetes, orthopedic surgeons have seen a greater percentage of their patients undergoing elective and posttraumatic foot and ankle surgery diagnosed with diabetes as well. It has been reported in one review of 160,000 patients with ankle fractures, 5.7% were diabetic.[2]

Diabetes also appears to dramatically increase the risk of lower extremity amputation because of infected, nonhealing foot ulcers.[3] The rates of amputation in diabetic populations are typically 10 to 20 times those of nondiabetic individuals, and over the past decade have ranged from 1.5 to 3.5 events per 1000 persons per year in populations with diagnosed diabetes.[1] Thus, orthopedic lower extremity surgeons are seeing a larger number of patients needing amputations than were encountered in previous decades.

Orthopedic surgeons who treat foot and ankle disorders must recognize the unique characteristics of diabetic patients to provide optimal care, and to ensure satisfactory outcomes. The physiologic and metabolic abnormalities seen in diabetic patients can adversely affect healing, even in the simplest of procedures. Neuropathy, vasculopathy, and altered tissue healing are very common in diabetic patients, and can negatively affect surgical treatments. Operative treatment has a higher complication rate in diabetic patients versus normoglycemic patients, especially in

---

Disclosure Statement: No relevant commercial or financial conflicts of interest. Per the American Academy of Orthopaedic Surgeons (AAOS) disclosure statement, these conflicts have been reported- Board member/committee member for a society- AAOS Board of Councilors, Florida Orthopedic Society Board of Directors, American Orthopaedic Foot & Ankle Society Fellowship Match Committee; Reviewer for Foot and Ankle International; Paid lecturer for Arthrex, Inc.

[a] Tallahassee Orthopedic Clinic, 3334 Capital Medical Boulevard, Tallahassee, FL 32308, USA; [b] Florida State University College of Medicine, 1115 W Call Street, Tallahassee, FL 32304, USA; [c] Alabama College of Osteopathic Medicine, 445 Health Sciences Boulevard, Dothan, AL 36303, USA; [d] Tallahassee Memorial Hospital, 1300 Miccosukee Road, Tallahassee, FL 32308, USA
* Tallahassee Orthopedic Clinic, 3334 Capital Medical Boulevard, Tallahassee, FL 32308.
E-mail address: aaron.guyer@tlhoc.com

those who have common comorbidities, such as peripheral neuropathy and peripheral vascular disease.[2,4–8] This article examines some of the special considerations in the treatment of diabetic patients undergoing foot and ankle surgeries.

PHYSIOLOGIC AND METABOLIC CONSIDERATIONS

Many diabetic patients incorrectly believe that the only problem with their disease is they have "high sugar." Diabetes affects many physiologic and metabolic systems of the body, and therefore, many organ systems. As a result, there are multiple aspects of healing that can be affected by the disease.

Hemoglobin A1C levels (HgBA1C) are a well-known measure of diabetic glycemic control. Although an elevated value has not been directly linked to complications, patients with higher HgBA1C are more likely to have end-stage complications of diabetes, such as vascular disease and neuropathy, which can significantly affect surgical outcomes.[8] All patients with known diabetes should have a HgBA1C level measured before any elective surgical procedure, as should those with acute traumatic injuries. Ideally, HgBA1C levels should be less than or equal to 8 before embarking on any elective foot and ankle surgeries in diabetic patients, as levels greater than this have been associated with a higher rate of mechanical hardware failures, infection, and other morbidity.[4] Perioperative glucose levels also should be monitored, as previous research has demonstrated a higher risk of infection and healing problems in patients who remain hyperglycemic during this time.[5]

Diabetes causes multiple abnormalities in immune system function as well. Leukocyte chemotaxis, adherence, phagocytosis, and intracellular killing, all integral to infection response, are negatively affected by diabetes.[7] As a result, diabetic patients have an 80% higher risk of cellulitis, a fourfold greater risk of osteomyelitis, and twofold increased risk of sepsis and death, as compared with nondiabetic individuals.[6] In addition, a diabetic patient's physiologic response to infection is slowed compared with other patients. Diabetic patients will elicit a fever and increased white blood cell count less often than nondiabetic individuals, which is likely due to impaired immune response. One of the earliest signs of infection has been noted to be worsening glycemic control, and this has been used previously in diabetic patients to differentiate moderate from severe infection.[9] A surgeon operating on diabetic patients should keep these factors in mind, and be vigilant in recognizing and aggressively treating even the first suspected signs of infection. The judicious use of antibiotics, as well as early irrigation and debridement of suspected postoperative infections, can decrease the chance of deep infection and further morbidity.

CONTRIBUTION OF NEUROPATHY

Peripheral neuropathy has been found to be one of the most important concomitant risk factors of diabetes associated with surgical complications.[6,7,10,11] It is estimated that there is an 8% incidence of neuropathy at the time of diagnosis, but this can increase up to 50% at 25 years after diagnosis.[6] Neuropathies proceed in a stocking-glove manner from distal to proximal.

Although diabetes affects all nerve types, sensory neuropathy is the most common, and affects up to 75% of patients. Loss of protective sensation can lead to skin breakdown due to repetitive trauma, ultimately causing ulcers and infection. Diagnosis of peripheral neuropathy is initially made on physical examination, with 5.07 Semmes-Weinstein monofilament testing. This is considered to be the minimum threshold at which protective sensation is intact, and loss of sensation at this level is thought to be associated with the development of neuropathic pressure ulcers and Charcot neuroarthropathy.[7] Evaluation of a diabetic patient undergoing either elective or posttraumatic foot and ankle surgeries should include this monofilament testing of sensation. Suspected peripheral neuropathy from physical examination findings also can be confirmed with nerve conduction studies/electromyography.

Motor neuropathy can lead to foot deformities, such as claw toes and hammer toes. These deformities, especially once they become rigid, produce pressure points where shoes, casts, and braces can rub and result in ulcerations, particularly in patients who also have sensory neuropathy. Additionally, pain and temperature sensation can become diminished, as can vibratory perception. Up to 30% of patients with peripheral neuropathy also will report neuropathic pain, described as burning, shooting, cramping, "electrical," or tingling.

Autonomic disturbances have multiple effects, including skin changes, vascular dysregulation, and loss of proprioception, which contributes to the development of Charcot arthropathy. The loss of sweat production and blood vessel tone causes skin to become dry, cracked, and fissured, which contributes to the development of cellulitis and provides a portal for infection risk.

Charcot arthropathy affects fewer than 1% of all diabetic patients, but up to 13% of high-risk patients with diabetes.[6] Although there are multiple cause of this neuroarthropathy, diabetes mellitus remains the most common etiology worldwide.[8] The pathophysiology of Charcot arthropathy is complex, but is believed to ultimately stem from the autonomic dysregulation of vasculature, combined with repetitive microtrauma resulting from loss of normal mechanoreception. Localized osteopenia results from altered blood flow to the foot, and thus makes bones more susceptible to fracture. As a result, massive joint and bone destruction results, sometimes with an apparently minor traumatic injury. Many patients present without significant pain, only with swelling, warmth, and deformity, which sometimes mimics infection. Diagnosis can be made by physical examination, as well as on radiographs showing severe bone destruction and joint collapse. Differentiating Charcot arthropathy from infection can be difficult, as both conditions can present similarly. There are several key features of Charcot arthropathy, however, that can help a clinician distinguish between these 2 very different diagnoses. The swelling, erythema, and warmth decreases with elevation of the limb in neuroarthropathy, but it does not in infection. Infection is less likely, and neuroarthropathy more likely, in the absence of an open wound or ulcer, and with no change in recent glycemic control. MRI and computed tomography scan generally are not helpful, as osteomyelitis and Charcot arthropathy look very similar on these studies. Bone scan combined with Indium 111–labeled white blood cell scans can often assist in making the diagnosis, but can take up to a week for the results of the study to be available.

It is important to recognize Charcot changes in diabetic patients undergoing both elective and posttraumatic surgeries. The surgical approach, operative timing, and type of fixation are all very different for patients demonstrating neuroarthropathic changes and those who do not. Failure to identify Charcot features can lead to an increased rate of wound-healing and bone-healing complications, which ultimately could result in amputation. Traditionally, surgical timing in patients with Charcot arthropathy has been based on what healing phase a patient demonstrates. According to the Eichenholtz classification, there are 3 temporal stages of Charcot neuropathy. Stage I is the "development" or "fragmentation" stage, characterized clinically by hyperemia, swelling, erythema, and warmth. Radiographically, there is joint dislocation and fracture. This phase may last 2 to 4 months. Stage II, or the "coalescence" phase, demonstrates new bone formation on radiographs, and decreased warmth and erythema on physical examination. Finally, stage III, or "consolidation," demonstrates healed fractures with residual clinical deformity but no further warmth or erythema. The deformity tends to be stable at this point, although it can slowly progress occasionally.[12] Ideally, the consolidation (inactive) stage of Charcot arthropathy has been reached before any foot or ankle surgery, and is associated with lower complication rates. Protected weightbearing in total contact casts or bracing should be used during stages I and II. The exception is in ankle neuroarthropathy, in which significant malalignment can develop quickly and compromise the soft tissue envelope. These ankle deformities are also difficult to brace, and early arthrodesis may be optimal. Close observation of skin condition and deformity magnitude is paramount in such patients to ensure a satisfactory outcome.[13]

VASCULOPATHY

The incidence of peripheral vascular disease is 30 times more common in diabetic patients than other patient populations.[6] Therefore, it is essential that the vascular status of diabetic patients undergoing elective or posttraumatic surgeries be thoroughly evaluated preoperatively. If a patient's dorsalis pedis and posterior tibial pulses are not palpable on physical examination, the use of a handheld Doppler should be used to confirm major vessel flow to the foot. Ankle Brachial Index (ABI) testing alone can be unreliable in diabetic patients, as calcification of vessels may give false-negative results. Toe pressures or transcutaneous oxygen pressure are other tests that can be used to evaluate distal foot perfusion, and are thought to be more reliable than ABI alone.[7] Wukich and colleagues[14] recently examined combining Toe Brachial Index (TBI) and great toe pressures with ABI as a screening tool for peripheral artery disease. They concluded that TBI was more reliable than ABI alone in diagnosing vascular disease in the diabetic population, and that both ABI and TBI should be used as a noninvasive measure of peripheral perfusion. If there is any question of adequate blood flow to the foot or ankle, a vascular surgery consult should be obtained, as angiography may be required to fully confirm arterial lesions. Revascularization procedures may be needed before treating both elective and posttraumatic foot and ankle problems surgically, to ensure adequate perfusion to healing bone and soft tissues.

HEALING CONSIDERATIONS

The physiologic and metabolic abnormalities seen in diabetic patients can negatively affect both bone and soft tissue healing following surgery. Delayed bony unions or nonunions, and delayed skin healing, unfortunately, are all too common in diabetic surgical patients.

Multiple aspects of bone healing are negatively affected in diabetes. The strength of fracture callus is decreased in diabetic patients, length of time to healing is prolonged, and mechanical stiffness of healing bone is lower.[7] Bone-healing complications have been found to be significantly associated with peripheral neuropathy, elevated HgBA1C, and longer surgery durations. One series of 165 patients demonstrated that neuropathy was the most significant risk factor for bone-healing complications.[10] Therefore, all diabetic patients should be screened for peripheral neuropathy as well as adequate glycemic control as elucidated from a recent HgBA1C. Due to longer healing times and biomechanically weaker bone, non-weightbearing immobilization following orthopedic surgery should be prolonged, and consideration should be given to more rigid, and sometimes additional, fixation.

Wound complications are higher in diabetic patients than nondiabetic individuals, and wounds also take longer to heal. The soft tissue envelope should be carefully evaluated before any surgical interventions, especially in posttraumatic patients. Severe swelling, evidence of chronic venous stasis, and dry, cracking, inelastic skin, are all harbingers of poor wound healing postoperatively.[8] Preoperatively, edema control is essential, and often in posttraumatic patients, surgery may need to be delayed longer than usual to ensure adequate soft tissue condition. Postoperatively, vigilant wound management is needed, to ensure satisfactory outcomes. In comparison with normoglycemic patients, diabetic patients may require more frequent dressing changes, wound evaluations, and prolonged postoperative suture retention.

Glycemic control has been shown to be one of the most important factors in preventing postsurgical complications, as well as improving healing. The Diabetes Control and Complications Research Trial Group demonstrated that intensive glycemic control delays the onset and slows the progression of diabetic retinopathy, nephropathy, and neuropathy in patients with diabetes.[15] This is particularly important in surgical patients, as patients with these comorbidities have far more complications than those diabetic patients

without such diagnoses. More recently, in a prospective study, Wukich and colleagues[11] examined surgical site infection incidence following foot and ankle surgery. Their analysis demonstrated that peripheral neuropathy and an HgBA1C of ≥8% were independently associated with surgical site infection 2.7 times greater than patients with HgBA1C less than 8%. Another series examined 348 diabetic patients undergoing elective foot and ankle surgery at a single institution. Those with blood glucose levels ≥200 mg/dL in the perioperative period were found to have a 2.45% higher rate of surgical site infections than those who were maintained at levels below 200.[5] Hence, the investigators recommended consultation with internal medicine consultants in all diabetic patients undergoing elective foot and ankle surgeries to maintain strict glycemic control. These studies demonstrate the importance of tight glycemic control in patients undergoing foot and ankle surgeries, both long-term control and in the perioperative period.

ANKLE FRACTURES IN DIABETIC PATIENTS

Ankle fractures are one of the most common injuries that orthopedic surgeons treat, and many of the principles used in treating diabetic patients with ankle fractures also can be applied to other elective or semi-elective orthopedic procedures in this patient population.

Diabetic patients with ankle fractures have a much higher rate of morbidity and complications associated with both nonoperative and operative treatments. These include delayed wound healing, infection, loss of fixation, delayed union or nonunion, and Charcot arthropathy. Because of this higher rate of operative complications, surgeons may feel inclined to treat these fractures in a closed fashion. Poor results have not been limited to operatively treated fractures, however, in diabetic patients. Several studies have demonstrated up to a 66% incidence of infection and a 70% risk of malunion in ankle fractures treated closed with casting.[16] In addition, a recent study by Lovy and colleagues,[17] demonstrated that nonoperative treatment for displaced ankle fractures in diabetic patients actually had a higher complication rate than a similar cohort of patients treated operatively. This retrospective study of 20 patients treated nonoperatively showed a 75% rate of complications, including malunion, loss of reduction, new-onset Charcot arthropathy, cast ulcers, deep infection, and unplanned subsequent operation, compared with surgical treatment. The operative group demonstrated only a

12.5% rate of similar complications. Previous studies have shown similar complication rates with nonoperatively treated displaced ankle fractures in diabetic populations.[18,19] Therefore, operative fixation should be considered as primary treatment for any displaced ankle fracture that would be treated with open reduction internal fixation (ORIF) in a nondiabetic individual.

Operative indications for treating ankle fractures should be considered the same for diabetic patients and nondiabetic individuals. Fractures that are nondisplaced and considered stable can be treated nonoperatively; however, they require vigilant follow-up and prolonged non-weightbearing, even up to 6 months' duration. Total Contact Casting is often needed in neuropathic patients to prevent cast ulcerations, and to improve immobilization of the injured limb. Displaced and unstable injuries should be treated with standard operative techniques. There are several principles, however, that need to be applied to this patient population to achieve a satisfactory result and avoid complications.

A thorough physical examination is an essential part of any evaluation in patients presenting with an ankle fracture. The high rate of comorbidities in diabetic patients necessitates careful preoperative evaluation. Like normoglycemic patients, diabetic patients with ankle fractures will present with swelling, deformity, ecchymosis, and tenderness over the fracture site. Open wounds, significant swelling, and fracture blisters can all lead to wound-healing problems in any patient, but can be especially devastating for diabetic individuals, given their higher propensity to infection and delayed wound healing. Dry, cracked, atrophic, or thin skin commonly found in diabetic patients can increase the chance of cellulitis or deep infection developing. Based on soft tissue envelope findings, more immediate reduction and provisional fixation may be needed to prevent skin pressure sores from displaced ankle fractures. Conversely, those patients without impending skin compromise but who have massive swelling, may require delayed surgical intervention until soft tissue conditions improve. Neurologic and vascular evaluation is also essential to identify patients with peripheral neuropathy and vasculopathy, as both of these disorders are common in the diabetic population, and associated with a higher rate of postoperative complications. All patients with diminished sensation should be screened with 5.07 Semmes-Weinstein monofilament testing. Nonpalpable pulses should be further evaluated with noninvasive testing, including Doppler, toe pressures, or transcutaneous oxygen levels. Some patients may require vascular surgery consult and intervention before ORIF if there is any suspicion of significant preexisting peripheral vascular disease.

Every diabetic patient considered for operative fixation should undergo preoperative laboratory evaluation, including both a current blood glucose level and an HgBA1C level. Acutely elevated glucose levels have been associated with higher infection risk in the perioperative period.[4,11] Chronically poor glycemic control increases the chances of neuropathy, vascular disease, and nephropathy, all of which can complicate wound and bone healing, and has been associated with a higher rate of surgical site infections.[8,11]

Identification of patients with Charcot arthropathy is essential in guiding operative techniques. Diabetic patients who initially present with massive swelling, warmth, deformity, or radiographic features suggestive of neuroarthropathy may require augmented fixation, or even primary arthrodesis. Those without these features can be treated according to standard fixation principles, but may need additional hardware to account for the poor bone quality and prolonged time required for union. Multiple syndesmotic screw supplementation (often referred to as "the ladder") can increase rigidity of lateral ankle fixation (**Fig. 1**). Adding transarticular large Steinman pins can keep the ankle joint reduced while the fracture sites medially, laterally, and posteriorly are healing (**Fig. 2**). Locking plates can increase biomechanical stiffness in osteopenic bone as well. External fixation augmentation also may be needed to stabilize highly unstable diabetic ankle fractures (**Fig. 3**).

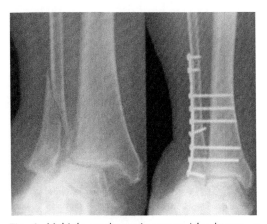

Fig. 1. Multiple syndesmotic screws (also known as "the ladder") can be used to improve stability of fibula fractures. (*From* Johnson JE, Klein SE, Brodsky JW. Diabetes. In: Coughlin MJ, Saltzman CL, Anderson RB, editors. Mann's surgery of the foot and ankle. 9th edition. Philadelphia: Saunders, an imprint of Elsevier Inc; 2014. p. 1471; with permission.)

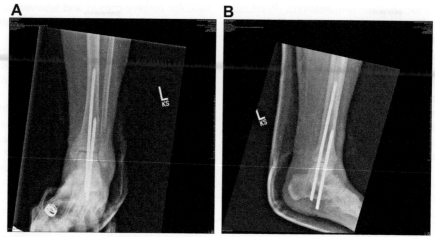

Fig. 2. (A, B) Transarticular large Steinman pins can keep an ankle joint reduced in patients with poor bone quality, poor skin condition, or in highly unstable fractures.

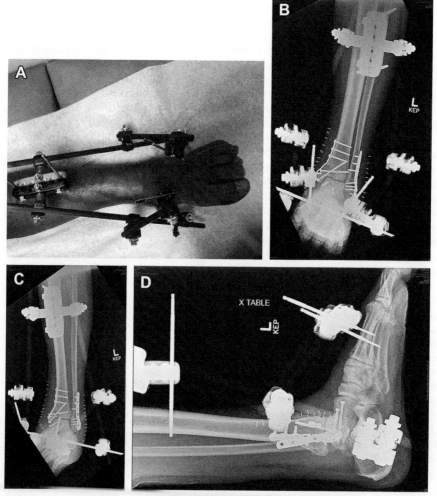

Fig. 3. (A–D) External fixation used to supplement fixation in a highly unstable bimalleolar ankle fracture.

Some diabetic patients may require less-invasive surgical treatment and fixation than that used in nondiabetic patients, due to severe swelling, poor soft tissue envelope condition, or other medical comorbidities that would risk complications. Closed reduction, or open reduction with small incisions can be used, followed by fixation with K-wires, external fixation, or transarticular Steinmann pins in this population. Intramedullary fibula rods and cannulated screws are other types of hardware that also can be inserted via small incisions.

SUMMARY

Foot and ankle surgery in the diabetic population can be challenging. Although the complication rate is higher than in normoglycemic patients, satisfactory outcomes can be achieved if surgeons are vigilant in identifying and managing common comorbidities, and if several special principles are adhered to.

REFERENCES

1. World Health Organization. Global report on diabetes, vol. 978. Isbn; 2016. p. 88. ISBN 978 92 4 156525 7.
2. Ganesh SP, Pietrobon R, Cecílio WA, et al. The impact of diabetes on patient outcomes after ankle fracture. J Bone Joint Surg Am 2005;87(8):1712–8.
3. Moxey PW, Gogalniceanu P, Hinchliffe RJ, et al. Lower extremity amputations—a review of global variability in incidence. Diabet Med 2011;28(10):1144–53.
4. Wukich DK, Lowery NJ, McMillen RL, et al. Postoperative infection rates in foot and ankle surgery: a comparison of patients with and without diabetes mellitus. J Bone Joint Surg Am 2010;92(2):287–95.
5. Sadoskas D, Suder N, Wukich D. Perioperative glycemic control and the effect on surgical site infections in diabetic patients undergoing foot and ankle surgery. Foot Ankle Spec 2015;3(1):15–20.
6. Thomas R. Diabetic foot disease. In: Chou L, editor. Orthopaedic knowledge update 5, foot and ankle. Rosemont (IL): American Academy of Orthopaedic Surgeons; 2014. p. 67–83.
7. Ishikawa S. Diabetic foot. In: Canale S, Beaty J, editors. Campbell's operative orthopaedics. 12th

edition. Philadelphia: Elsevier Mosby; 2013. p. 4057–77.
8. Johnson JE, Klein SE, Brodsky JW. Diabetes. In: Coughlin M, Saltzman C, Anderson R, editors. Mann's surgery of the foot and ankle. 9th edition. Philadelphia: Elsevier Saunders; 2014. p. 1385–480.
9. Wukich DK, Hobizal KB, Brooks MM. Severity of diabetic foot infection and rate of limb salvage. Foot Ankle Int 2013;34(3):351–8.
10. Shibuya N, Humphers JM, Fluhman BL, et al. Factors associated with nonunion, delayed union, and malunion in foot and ankle surgery in diabetic patients. J Foot Ankle Surg 2013;52(2):207–11.
11. Wukich DK, Crim BE, Frykberg RG, et al. Neuropathy and poorly controlled diabetes increase the rate of surgical site infection after foot and ankle surgery. J Bone Joint Surg Am 2014;96(10):832–9.
12. Rosenbaum AJ, DiPreta JA. Classifications in brief: Eichenholtz classification of Charcot arthropathy. Clin Orthop Relat Res 2014;473(3):1168–71.
13. Wukich DK, Raspovic KM, Hobizal KB, et al. Surgical management of Charcot neuroarthropathy of the ankle and hindfoot in patients with diabetes. Diabetes Metab Res Rev 2016;32:292–6.
14. Wukich DK, Shen W, Raspovic KM, et al. Noninvasive arterial testing in patients with diabetes: a guide for foot and ankle surgeons. Foot Ankle Int 2015;36(12):1391–9.
15. The Diabetes Control and Complications Trial Research Group. The effect of intensive treatment of diabetes on the development and progression of long-term complications in insulin-dependent diabetes mellitus. N Engl J Med 1993;329(14): 977–86.
16. Flynn JM, Rio FR, Pizá PA. Closed ankle fractures in the diabetic patient. Foot Ankle Int 2000;21(4): 311–9.
17. Lovy AJ, Dowdell J, Keswani A, et al. Nonoperative versus operative treatment of displaced ankle fractures in diabetics. Foot Ankle Int 2017;38(3): 255–60.
18. Schon LC, Easley ME, Weinfeld SB. Charcot neuroarthropathy of the foot and ankle. Clin Orthop Relat Res 1998;349:116–31.
19. McCormack RG, Leith JM. Ankle fractures in diabetics. Complications of surgical management. J Bone Joint Surg Br 1998;80(4):689–92.

Moving?

Make sure your subscription moves with you!

To notify us of your new address, find your **Clinics Account Number** (located on your mailing label above your name), and contact customer service at:

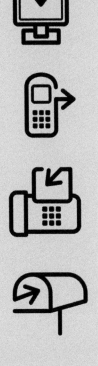

Email: journalscustomerservice-usa@elsevier.com

800-654-2452 (subscribers in the U.S. & Canada)
314-447-8871 (subscribers outside of the U.S. & Canada)

Fax number: 314-447-8029

Elsevier Health Sciences Division
Subscription Customer Service
3251 Riverport Lane
Maryland Heights, MO 63043

*To ensure uninterrupted delivery of your subscription, please notify us at least 4 weeks in advance of move.

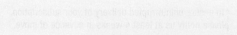

Printed and bound by CPI Group (UK) Ltd, Croydon, CR0 4YY

08/05/2025

01864713-0009